# Handbook of
## Patient Transport

# Handbook of
# Patient Transportation

**T. E. Martin** MB BS, DAvMed, FIMC, FRCS
Specialist Registrar in Anaesthetics
John Radcliffe Hospital, Oxford

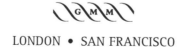

LONDON • SAN FRANCISCO

Greenwich Medical Media Limited
137 Euston Road
London NW1 2AA

870 Market Street, Ste 720,
San Francisco, CA 94102

ISBN 1 84110 071 4

First Published 2001

A catalogue record for this book is available from the British Library.

Project Manager
Gavin Smith

Typeset by Charon Tec Pvt. Ltd, Chennai, India

Printed in the UK by Alden Press

Distributed by Plymbridge Distributors Ltd and
in the USA by Jamco Distribution

Visit our website at www.greenwich-medical.co.uk

# Contents

# Preface

*Ambulance.* The word conjures up a vision of a gleaming white vehicle rushing past with lights flashing and sirens blaring. On board, EMTs, paramedics, and may be even a doctor or nurse, are battling to save the life of an unfortunate victim of trauma, or of sudden unexpected illness. But the word originally referred to movement (from *ambulare*, Latin for 'to walk' or 'to move'), and it has only become associated with emergency transportation of patients since the Napoleonic Wars.

The scope of this book is wide. There is clearly a great dissimilarity between the operations of an urban paramedic road ambulance, and an air ambulance which specializes only in long-distance repatriations. This is not to mention the disparity between those of a doctor organizing an intrahospital transfer of an ITU patient to, say, a remote MRI scanner, and of an ambulance technician who has been called to an elderly collapsed patient at home. Similarly, the reader may be forgiven for searching for some connection between the relatively healthy postoperative patient who may require only a nurse escort from his holiday destination to home, and the critically injured child who is airlifted, unconscious and bleeding, from the scene of a RTA. However, this book details the major principles of patient transportation and discusses the special needs of each of these environments. It is a practically based text in which the reader will find easy-to-digest details on clinical management and on the logistics of different transport modes as well as facts about the physics and physiology of patient movement.

Units of measurement in the text are those most often used in either the medical or the transport (especially aviation) fraternity, not necessarily their Systéme Internationale equivalents. Drug names are given as generics and, to avoid the cumbersome use of multiple nouns, pronouns and adjectives, the male gender ('man', 'he', 'him', 'his') is used when, clearly, the text may refer to either sex.

The text is intended as a primer and handbook for those who work in transportation medicine, not just doctors, but also nurses, paramedics and those who administer ambulance and air ambulance organizations. It contains a fascinating mix of physics and physiology, of aeronautics, and of clinical care, but a book of this size cannot be a definitive text and does not aim to be.

Finally a word of caution about undertaking the transfer that just does not quite feel right. For each individual, the problem is understanding one's own limitations and being aware of the potential pitfalls that lay ahead. Hopefully this book will grant you the knowledge and comfort to set out in confidence, and yet to postpone your transfer or to seek senior help when warning bells sound. If a problem can occur in transport, it probably will.

TEM
January 2001

# Acknowledgements

I am indebted to the following individuals and organizations who kindly provided information or materials for the text: The Welsh Ambulance Service, Mid Glamorgan; First Air, Cornwall & Isles of Scilly Ambulance Service; London Helicopter Emergency Medical Service; Europ Assistance, London; AEA (now International SOS), Singapore; Tactical Medical Wing, Royal Air Force Lyneham; Dr Tania Abreu and Dr Fiona Jewkes.

T. E. Martin
January 2001

# Abbreviations

| | |
|---|---|
| AA | Automobile Association |
| ABC | Airway, breathing, and circulation |
| ACLS | Advanced cardiac life support |
| ALS | Advanced life support |
| ATLS | Advanced trauma life support |
| BASICS | British Association of Immediate Care (Schemes) |
| BP | Blood pressure |
| BSA | Body surface area |
| CAA | Civil Aviation Authority |
| CCU | Coronary care unit |
| CNS | Central nervous system |
| $CO_2$ | Carbon dioxide |
| CPAP | Continuous positive airway pressure |
| CPP | Cerebral perfusion pressure |
| CPR | Cardiopulmonary resuscitation |
| CSF | Cerebrospinal fluid |
| CT | Computerized tomography scan(ner) |
| CVP | Central venous pressure |
| DCS | Decompression sickness |
| DNR | Do not resuscitate |
| DVT | Deep vein thrombosis |

| ECG | Electrocardiograph(y) |
|---|---|
| EMS | Emergency medical services |
| EMT | Emergency medical technician |
| ERC | European Resuscitation Council |
| $FIO_2$ | Inspired oxygen concentration |
| G | Unit of gravitational acceleration |
| GCS | Glasgow Coma Score (or Scale) |
| GP | General practioner |
| Hb | Haemoglobin |
| HbF | Foetal haemoglobin |
| HEMS | Helicopter emergency medical service |
| HR | Heart rate |
| IABC | Intra-aortic balloon counterpulsation |
| ICP | Intracranial pressure |
| ICU | Intensive care unit |
| IHR | International Health Regulation |
| ITU | Intensive therapy unit |
| IV | Intravenous |
| LOX | Liquid oxygen |
| MAST | Medical (or military) antishock trousers |
| MEDIF | Medical information form |
| MRI | Magnetic resonance imaging scan(ner) |
| MV | Minute volume |
| NAAS | National Association of Air Ambulance System |
| NG | Nasogastric |
| NHS | National Health Service (UK) |
| NICU | Neonatal intensive care unit |
| ODA/ODP | Operating department assistant/practitioner |
| PASG | Pneumatic antishock garment |
| $PCO_2$ | Partial pressure of carbon dioxide |
| PE | Pulmonary embolism |
| PEEP | Positive end expiratory pressure |
| PHTLS | Prehospital trauma life support |
| PICU | Paediatric intensive care unit |

| | |
|---|---|
| $PO_2$ | Partial pressure of oxygen |
| psi | Pounds per square inch |
| RAF | Royal Air Force |
| RNLI | Royal National Lifeboat Institute |
| RTA | Road traffic accident |
| SAMU | Service d'Aide Medicale Urgente |
| SAR | Search and Rescue |
| SCBU | Special care baby unit |
| SIMV | Synchronized intermittent mandatory ventilation |
| SV | Stroke volume |

# Contributors

**Terry Martin** MB BS, DAvMed, FIMC, FRCS
Specialist Registrar in Anaesthetics
John Radcliffe Hospital, Oxford

**Juergen Rayner-Klein** FIMC, FRCA
Consultant in Anaesthesia and Intensive Care Medicine
Southern Derbyshire Acute Hospitals, NHS Trust

**Fiona Jewkes** MB ChB, FRCP, FRCPCH
Consultant Paediatrician
University Hospital of Wales, Cardiff

**Jonathan Warwick** MB ChB, FRCA
Consultant Anaesthetist
Radcliffe Infirmary, Oxford

# 1

# Overview of medical transportation

Until the early 20th century, ambulance vehicle development was led by the need for the removal of injured soldiers from battlefields, whereas in the past 50 years the increasing requirement to transfer patients is more dependent on the evolution of modern medical technology and on the economics of health care delivery.

Out-of-hospital medical transport may involve primary, secondary, or tertiary responses and patients are usually transferred to hospital by road ambulance, although this function may occasionally be undertaken by helicopter:

- *Primary responses* – the ambulance serves as the sole means of patient transport to a receiving facility. These 'scene missions' are usually of short duration.
- *Secondary responses* – vehicles or aircraft involved in secondary missions transfer patients from outlying emergency facilities where some degree of stabilization has been performed, to the care of a higher-level facility.
- *Tertiary responses* – when an ambulance or aircraft transports a hospital inpatient to another facility for specialist or definitive care, or when patients are repatriated after injury or illness sustained overseas.

- The use of ground vehicles and aircraft in the transport of medications, equipment, medical personnel, and human tissues or organ harvest teams represents yet another facet of medical transportation.

Once in the hospital, further transfers may be necessary. Modern medicine may dictate that the patient requires transport within the hospital (intrahospital) from the A&E department to

- an imaging scanner (such as computerized tomography (CT), angiography, or magnetic resonance imaging (MRI)),
- the operating theatre,
- a critical care unit (such as intensive therapy unit (ITU), paediatric intensive care unit (PICU), special care baby unit (SCBU), coronary care unit (CCU) or specialist intensive care).

## BEGINNINGS

### The military

- Battle wounded were tended and transported by early Greek and Roman soldiers.
- The concept of an ambulance service started during the Crusades of the 11th century.
- The Knights of St John were taught first aid by Arab and Greek doctors and then acted as the ambulance technicians of their day, treating soldiers at the point of wounding and transporting them to casualty collection points for further care.
- The French army created the first official medical corps in 1792.
- Trained attendants took equipment on to the battlefield and rendered first aid before transporting the wounded

back to the field hospitals by stretcher, hand-carts and wagons.

Baron Dominique Jean Larrey (1766–1842), Surgeon-in-Chief and a personal friend of Napoleon, has been credited with the establishment of these unique and advanced medical evacuation procedures. He recognized the value of bringing medical aid to the wounded and he developed a *triage* system to prioritize the order of treatment and evacuation. Inspired by the *artillene volant* (flying artillery), which closely followed the advanced guard, Larrey designed and produced several two- and four-wheeled carts and called them *ambulance volante* (flying ambulances). These were fast and manoeuverable like the artillery, but carried surgeons and their equipment to the battlefields, and then returned with the wounded to nearby field hospitals.

## Civilian history

- During the 19th century the police were called to accidents and cases of sudden illness.
- Hand stretchers were used to convey patients to hospital.
- Wheeled stretchers were introduced in 1880.
- Ambulance services for non-infectious patients were established in London and Glasgow in 1882.
- Evolving ambulance services relied almost exclusively on private benefactors.
- An Act of Parliament in England and Wales compelled local authorities to organize ambulance services.
- In 1948, under Section 27 of the newly introduced National Health Service (NHS) Act, it became the duty of local health authorities in England and Wales to provide ambulance services free of charge.
- The Scottish Ambulance Service was established by the union of the St Andrew's and Red Cross Ambulance

Services. They made their joint fleet available to the Secretary of State for Scotland.

Horse-drawn vehicles were in common use in Britain at the beginning of the 20th century. War was still a stimulus for the improvement of ambulance design and, during the Boer War, the Secretary of State for War offered a prize of £500 for the best new design. Since then, there has been continued change, not only in vehicles and equipment but also in understanding the effects of movement on patients.

Motorized ambulances were introduced into civilian practice in the UK in 1903, although as recently as the 1960s, ambulances were still designed with disregard for the effects of illness and injury. For the first time, clinical evidence showed that patients respond adversely to movement and that transport can influence mortality. Ambulances in use at the time were criticized for inadequate illumination, poor heating, excess vibration and high-noise levels. Ineffective vehicle identification made passage through traffic difficult and the journey was known to adversely affect the performance of cardiopulmonary resuscitation (CPR). Since then, remarkable changes in ambulance design and performance have occurred. Roles have evolved and new vehicles have been designed as mobile intensive care units (ICUs) and specialist vehicles for the carriage of everything from wheelchair patients to neonatal incubators. The first civilian organization to take specialist care out to the community was the Newcastle-upon-Tyne Obstetric Emergency Service, founded by Professor Farquhar Murray in 1935 who coined the term 'Flying Squad'.

## Interhospital transport

A 'physician accompanied transport system' was started in the Toronto General Hospital in 1953. It evolved to provide a level of patient care during transport as close as possible to that received in Toronto's newly established critical care facility (one of the first in the world). ICUs flourished over the next two decades and Australia led the way in specialist transfer vehicle design. The 1973 *EM-Care* ambulance offered a smooth ride, low loading, a centrally placed stretcher, ceiling mounted oxygen outlets, a ventilator attachment, and internal dimensions that allowed medical escorts to stand.

In France, the Service d'Aide Medicale Urgente (SAMU), first created in Toulouse in 1967, carries out primary and secondary transfers. Each of the 96 administrative territories in France are required to provide a SAMU unit, but the first UK system specifically developed for the transport of critically ill adults was established in Glasgow a year later. By the early 1990s, this group had transferred over 2,000 patients, approximately 95% of these by road ambulance. Only one death occurred in this series, but many studies have highlighted the hazards of interhospital transport of critically ill patients:

- Hypotension and hypertension have both been reported after ambulance transport and due to vibration.
- Vibration may also cause either hypertension or cardiovascular depression, depending on the dominant frequency.
- Transient hypertension and dysrhythmias are associated with sudden acceleration forces during the journey.
- Complications are minimal if patients are resuscitated adequately before transport and sedated effectively during movement.
- Inexperience in the management of patients who are critically ill is the dominant factor in the development of complications during transfer.

## ORIGINS OF AEROMEDICAL TRANSPORTATION

- The earliest recorded air evacuation of wounded casualties took place during the First World War in an unmodified French fighter plane.
- In 1917, John Flynn, a Presbyterian minister conceived the idea of combining radio, aviation, and medicine to produce a 'mantle of safety' across the Australian outback.
- This was the forerunner of the Royal Flying Doctor Service which remains a vital part of outback Australian life to this day.
- The Royal Air Force (RAF) first used aircraft in the casualty evacuation role in Somaliland, in 1919.
- Throughout the 1920s, the RAF operated an air ambulance service within a 100-mile radius of London.
- In 1933, the first UK civilian air ambulance service was instigated in the Scottish Isles.
- Long-distance, high-altitude aeromedical evacuation was pioneered by the German Luftwaffe during the Spanish Civil War (1936–1941).
- In the latter years of the Second World War, more than 90% of allied casualties were evacuated by air, mostly using the venerable DC3 Dakota (Douglas C47, Figure 1.1).
- In 1942, the US military began training flight transport personnel for the specific purpose of medical escort duties, and the first dedicated aeromedical unit was formed.

The history of the development of helicopters as air ambulances:

- This was of particular significance because of their ability to operate in confined spaces.
- A helicopter was first used as an air ambulance after an explosion on a US Navy destroyer off New York in January 1944 when blood plasma was flown to Manhattan.

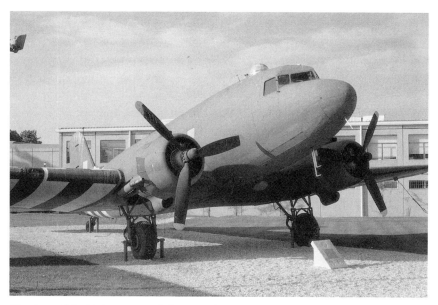

Fig. 1.1   DC3 Dakota – used for casualty evacuation in the Second World War.

- In April 1944, the same Coast Guard unit carried out the first air–sea rescue when a 15-year-old boy was airlifted from Jamaica Bay.
- In the late 1940s, helicopters were used in the casevac role by the British in Malaya.
- The first large-scale evacuation of wounded soldiers by helicopter occurred in Korea – over 20,000 wounded servicemen were transported strapped to stretchers outside the helicopter.

During the Vietnam War, over 400,000 patients were airlifted to hospital using dedicated squadrons of Bell UH-1 Iroquois ('Huey') aircraft (Figure 1.2). For the first time, casevac helicopters were used for the rapid removal of injured troops from close to the point of wounding. Casualties were then transported rapidly to nearby expert and specialist medical care for definitive treatment. This concept became known as 'scoop and run'.

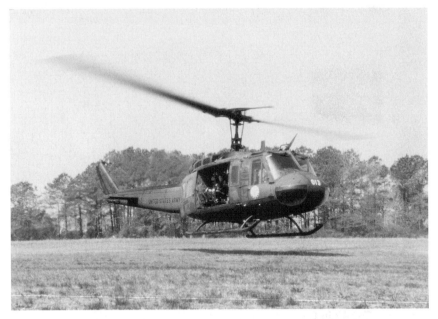

Fig. 1.2    Bell UH-1 Huey, first used in the casevac role in Vietnam.

## Civilian applications

Closely following the success of helicopters in Korea, a dramatic rescue occurred in New York during the summer of 1951. A steeplejack fell on to the roof of St John's Cathedral and refused to be lowered to the ground by ropes. Captain Gustav Crawford of the New York Police Aviation Bureau landed his helicopter on the roof of St John's and the casualty was strapped to the outside of the aircraft and flown to nearby Riverside Park where he was transported by ground ambulance to hospital.

In the 1960s, the immediacy of television news coverage on the Vietnam War brought public attention to the aeromedical helicopter and it was realized that the air ambulance might have an important contribution to make in civilian medical practice:

- Urban helicopters were first introduced in Maryland in 1969, to improve patient outcome in trauma – 'neglected disease of modern society'.

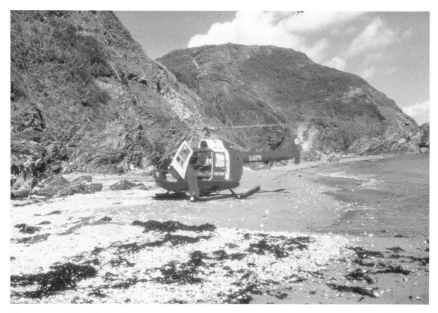

Fig. 1.3    *First Air* in Cornwall, England's first helicopter air ambulance (courtesy Cornwall & Isles of Scilly Ambulance Service).

- Four helicopters manned by paramedics were strategically stationed throughout the state for quick response to emergencies.
- The state-wide emergency medical services (EMS) system was designed by Dr William Cowley who originally coined the phrase 'The Golden Hour'.
- In the early 1980s, neonatal, obstetric, and cardiac air ambulance services were initiated in the USA.
- In the following two decades the number of interhospital flights have increased dramatically – 170 organizations were reported by 1992, and almost 200 in 1999.

The governments of Switzerland and Germany established combined military and civilian networks to cover all major highways and special risk areas such as large cities, coastline and mountainous terrain. In the UK, the 1980s saw the development of a paramedic crewed urban/coastal EMS helicopter (Figure 1.3) in Cornwall, soon followed by the London based helicopter emergency medical service (HEMS) which carries both a paramedic and doctor on every flight. Despite controversies over efficacy and costs, medical helicopter systems continue to proliferate, with 14 organizations operating in the EMS role in Great Britain:

- Cornwall
- Devon
- Kent
- Essex
- London
- Lincolnshire
- Nottinghamshire
- The West Midlands
- Northumbria
- Lancashire
- The Thames Valley
- Scotland
- Wales
- East Anglia

Some parts of the country still have no service at all, and in others the coverage is not 7 days a week. The Automobile Association (AA) has sponsored a new charity – the National Association of Air Ambulance Services (NAAS) – with an aim to help local charities to upgrade these systems, combined with a rolling programme to provide helicopters for areas not yet covered by 2002.

## Development of fixed-wing aeromedical services

The growth of international civil aeromedical transportation has been driven by rapid advances in the technology and availability of mass transportation. Larger and faster passenger carrying aircraft have brought cheap, affordable and accessible travel to millions of people throughout the world. Rapid airline growth in the post-war years and commercial exploitation have brought the most exotic corners of the Earth within reach of tourists and business travellers alike. Among these are a number who become ill or injured whilst abroad, some requiring repatriation

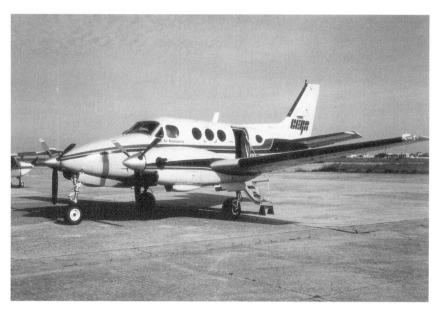

Fig. 1.4    Dedicated air ambulance.

on compassionate grounds, and others for specialist treatment. Numerous dedicated civilian medical assistance and air ambulance companies now exist (Figure 1.4). In the main, they operate in association with travel insurers, and arrange medical flights, worldwide, using fixed-wing aircraft.

## FURTHER READING

Bion IF, Wilson IH, Taylor PA (1988) Transporting critically ill patients by ambulance audit by sickness scoring. BMJ 296: 170.

Cleveland HC, Bigelow DB, Dracon D, Dustv F (1976) A civilian air emergency service: a report of its development, technical aspects, and experience. J Trauma 16: 452–463

Cook JL (1988) Dust Off. Rufus: New York.

Cullen CH, Douglas WK, Danziger AM (1967) Mortality of the ambulance ride. BMJ 3: 438.

Gabram SG, Jacobs LM (1990) The impact of emergency medical helicopters on prehospital care. Emer Med Clin North Am 8: 85–102.

London PS (1968) The design of ambulances. Proc Inst Mech Eng 182: I88.

Martin TE, Rodenberg HD (1996) Aeromedical Transportation: A Clinical Guide. Avebury: Aldershot.

National Academy of Sciences, National Research Council (1966), Accidental Death and Disability, the Neglected Disease of Modern Society, US Government Printing Office: Washington DC.

Neel SH (1968) Army aeromedical evacuation procedures in Vietnam. Implications for rural America. J Am Med Assoc 204: 99–103.

Pichard E (1970) The effect of acceleration and vibration on sick persons during transport. Rev Corps Sante 11: 611.

Snook R (1977) Transport of the injured patient past, present and future. Br J Anaesth 49: 651–658.

Snook R (1972) Medical aspects of ambulance design. BMJ 3: 574.

Wright IH, McDonald JC, Rogers PN, Ledingham IM (1988) Provision of facilities for secondary transport of seriously ill patients in the United Kingdom. BMJ 296(6621): 543–545.

# 2

# Physiology of patient movement

Very often little or no consideration is paid to the adverse effects of movement on the patient. Even for the fit and healthy, travel can be a tribulation. Vibration, for instance, can be irritating to the normal passenger but dangerous to the seriously ill patient, and it occurs in all forms of transport, not just in helicopters. Having said that, helicopters and fixed-wing aircraft (i.e. the flight environment) pose harsher conditions on the traveller, and the unwell passenger will suffer more. This chapter examines the major issues that are common to all forms of transport (vibration, motion sickness, noise and acceleration), and describes in some detail stresses particular to the flight environment (altitude and long haul flights). The so-called 'economy class syndrome' is not discussed since at this time there is no convincing evidence that deep vein thrombosis (DVT) and pulmonary embolism (PE) are *caused* by the flight environment, only that they are more likely to happen in susceptible individuals in whom venous stagnation occurs. This phenomenon is not restricted to the 'economy class', nor to flying, or even to travel. It is hoped that critically ill patients undertaking a long journey will already be in receipt of thromboprophylaxis.

## VIBRATION

Vibration and movement are constant and inevitable features of road and air travel:

- Vibration is alternating or oscillating forces that can be felt by the vehicle occupants.
- Vibration in land-based ambulances differs from that experienced in aircraft.
- The main source of vibration in road ambulances is the road surface and the vehicle's suspension system.
- The main source of vibration in fixed-wing aircraft is the engines and turbulence.
- Aircraft designers aim to minimize vibrations and ensure that any which can not be prevented will have minimum effect on the passengers and crew.
- Helicopters are a special case with vibration also caused by the gearbox, and main and tail rotors.

The most physiologically harmful frequencies lay between 0.1 and 40 Hz. Different body parts have natural frequencies, for instance the head resonates at about 6 Hz and the forearm at around 40 Hz. The problems include:

- Discomfort and fatigue as the passenger or patient uses muscular effort to stabilize the body.
- Low frequencies may cause blurred vision, shortness of breath, motion sickness, and chest or abdominal pain.
- Increased requirements for sedation and analgesia.
- Fracture sites may produce more discomfort.
- The pulse may be difficult to palpate.
- Interference with equipment, especially electronic monitoring systems and activity-sensing pacemakers.

- Sensors, electrodes and leads, like endotracheal tubes and intravenous lines, may easily become disconnected or dislodged.
- Automatic non-invasive blood pressure cuffs may fail to read.
- Gravity fed infusion devices become unreliable.
- Precision procedures, such as cannulation, may be impossible.

Nothing can be done by the medical escort to eliminate the vibration inherent in the vehicle, but the harmful and uncomfortable effects can be minimized by reduction of direct contact between the patient and the vehicle:

- Adequate energy-absorbing cushions, mattresses, or padding should be used for the stretcher and seats.
- Vehicle occupants should be firmly but comfortably restrained when vibration levels are high.

## NOISE

The vibration of air (sound) can be one of the most irritating factors encountered by medical personnel during patient transfers and excessive noise may interfere directly with patient care:

- Noise is sound which is loud or otherwise unpleasant.
- There is great individual variation in tolerance to its effects, and to what is considered unpleasant.
- The longer the exposure, and the more intense the noise, the greater the annoyance and inconvenience.
- Prolonged and intense exposure may also result in ear discomfort, deterioration in performance of tasks, headaches, fatigue, nausea, visual disturbances and vertigo.

Noise is generated by engines, road surfaces, the friction of air as it passes over the vehicle, aircraft propellers, helicopter rotors, radios, and medical monitoring equipment, in addition to any conversation generated by other people in the vehicle and the crew trying to communicate over the cacophony. A significant background level of noise renders the stethoscope useless and other means are required to monitor the patient:

- Visual observation of variations in respiratory rate, chest expansion, level of consciousness, and discomfort may be useful in monitoring the patient's respiratory condition.
- Blood pressure (BP) may be palpated or monitored by invasive or non-invasive devices.
- Further information can be gained from pulse oximetry and end-tidal capnography.

Noise produces other challenges for the medical team:

- Communication with an awake patient is difficult.
- Audible alarms may not be heard.
- Any change in tone of the pulse oximeter will not be apparent.
- Normal function of the ventilator (inspiratory/expiratory cycling) may not be heard.

Helicopter transportation is particularly noisy and hearing protection should be worn by both the medical crew and patient. Simple ear plugs or ear defenders will usually suffice, but head-sets offer better noise attenuation and will improve communications between crew members or between the patient and the medical team. The space between the noise attenuator, whatever is used, and the patient's tympanic membrane will become an external 'cavity' and will be subject to the problems of changes in gas volume with altitude.

## MOTION SICKNESS

Individuals vary in their response to motion stimuli and, although some may be very tolerant of the provocation caused by movement, if the stimulus is intense enough and of sufficient duration, all will eventually succumb. The mechanisms underlying the condition are not well understood, but motion sickness tends to happen when visual and vestibular evidence of motion are in conflict, or when signals from the semicircular canals and otoliths do not conform to expected patterns (*the sensory conflict theory*).

Infants are rarely air sick, but the incidence reaches a peak in late childhood and thereafter declines moderately with maturity. Women are more affected than men, and a number of factors are known to worsen or precipitate the symptoms:

- anxiety (general, or, indeed, a fear of being motion sick),
- unexpected motion,
- low-frequency oscillatory motion in the frequency range of 0.1–0.8 Hz,
- warm or stuffy environment,
- sight or smell of food,
- sight or smell of others vomiting,
- pre-existing nausea,
- gastric distension,
- ileus,
- nauseogenic medications.

Motion sickness is truly a debilitating experience and the signs and symptoms are probably familiar to every reader of this book. Sufferers may describe:

- increased 'stomach awareness',
- nausea,

- retching,
- vomiting,
- apathy, malaise, fatigue, or even exhaustion,
- a feeling of overwhelming warmth,
- headache,
- pallor and sweating.

Prevention in normal individuals:

- A sensible diet prior to transport.
- Victims may receive some comfort if their anxieties can be allayed, and if they are able to concentrate on an activity (although not reading, which tends to worsen the symptoms).
- Reducing sensory conflict, either by fixing the gaze outside of the vehicle, or by lying flat with the head still and the eyes closed.
- Anti-emetics for those known to be most susceptible.
- Many classes of drugs have been used, but none is significantly more effective than hyoscine (scopolamine).
- Most drugs have undesirable side effects that limit their use.
- Hyoscine causes drowsiness which is not improved when taken by transdermal route (skin patch).

Further management in patients whose condition may be worsened or compromised by vomiting – consider:

- Orogastric or nasogastric (NG) tube on free drainage.
- Anti-emetic polypharmacy (but not serotonin antagonists which have no effect in motion sickness).
- Ensure vomit bowls and a suction aspirator are nearby.
- Minimize movement.
- Any patient with wired or banded jaws should have cutting equipment immediately at hand.

## ACCELERATION

### The effects of acceleration

The Earth's gravitational envelope exposes us to an acceleration directed towards the centre of the planet with a magnitude of $32\,\text{ft/s}^2$, i.e. the 1G (multiples of $g$, the acceleration due to gravity) environment:

- This gravitational pull results in the force we know as weight.
- Modern transport can expose us to greater accelerations which may have profound physiological effects.
- Long-duration accelerations (several seconds in excess of 1G), add to the weight of objects and result in physiological changes as body organs and fluids obey Newton's third law of motion and respond with an equal and opposite reaction to the applied acceleration.
- Short-duration accelerations (less than 1 s duration, e.g. during a crash) very often result in injury or death.

### Long-duration acceleration

Although these accelerations occur in land vehicles, they are more troublesome in aircraft. Two types of acceleration may be experienced, linear and radial:

#### Linear acceleration

Linear acceleration results from an increase or decrease in the rate of movement along a straight line (Figure 2.1). No physiological consequences occur in the normal seated individual when the force is applied across the anteroposterior axis of the body (the actual direction depending on which way the occupant is seated) but stretcher patients lying parallel to the long axis of the aircraft are at risk of shift of body organs and fluid volumes

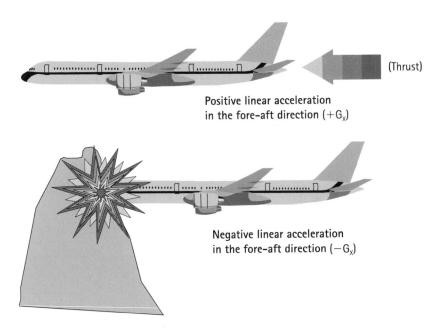

(Thrust)

Positive linear acceleration
in the fore–aft direction $(+G_x)$

Negative linear acceleration
in the fore–aft direction $(-G_x)$

Fig. 2.1   Linear acceleration.

in response to the inertial forces of linear acceleration. Blood
movement towards the lower extremities incites baroreceptor
reflexes with subsequent transient tachycardia in normal sub-
jects. There is debate over which way patients should travel, i.e.
head or foot first, but no clear evidence that transient changes
in cardiac output or intracranial pressure are important. In reality
few problems are seen and the logistics of patient loading usually limit the options. In most road and helicopter ambulances
the patient's head will be forward, but many fixed-wing air
ambulances adopt a foot first position arguing that it is safer
from a crash restraint point of view.

### Radial acceleration

Most commonly experienced in aircraft which have freedom of
movement in three axes, radial acceleration is due to a change
in direction of motion (Figure 2.2). The force acts outward from
the centre of a circular path but is perceived as an increase in
weight by the occupant. Acceleration is measured in G units

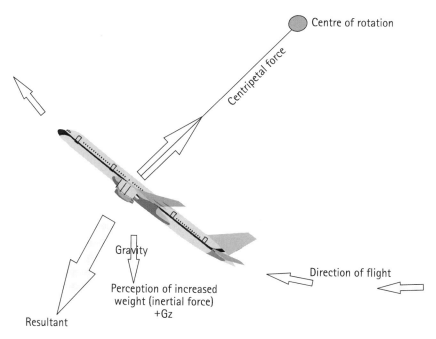

**Fig. 2.2   Radial acceleration.**

which, by convention, is labelled $G_z$ when the force acts in the long axis of the seated body, $G_x$ when it acts anteroposteriorly across the body, or $G_y$ when it acts laterally across the body. Positive acceleration with the head directed towards the centre of rotation ($+G_z$) is the force most commonly experienced. If $+G_z$ is sustained, the hydrostatic pressure in vessels below the level of the heart is increased and venous return is impaired. By Starling's law, cardiac output will follow, setting in train physiological responses resembling those seen in hypovolaemic states. Reflex tachycardia and selective vasoconstriction ensue in an attempt to maintain adequate blood pressure. At low levels of acceleration the hydrostatic effects are minimal and unlikely to be a serious cause for concern. Any patient with impaired circulation is already likely to be lying supine on a stretcher (with the acceleration now acting across the anteroposterior axis of the body). Medical crew should remember that the effect on weight is experienced by everything in the aircraft.

Consequently, traction weights, and monitors or equipment boxes resting on the patient will become heavier as the aircraft manoeuvres.

## TEMPERATURE

Consider the temperature of the patient's destination, as well as of the likely influences during the transfer. If departing a warm environment but expecting to arrive at night or in a cooler environment, take extra blankets or clothes. Some clinical conditions can exacerbate or cause hypothermia, such as hypothyroidism, spinal trauma or a major burn injury. Hypothermic patients should usually be warmed before a planned transfer is initiated.

The transport mode itself can affect thermoregulation:

- Exposure to moderate vibration results in a slight increase in metabolic rate.
- Vibration may also interfere with normal body thermoregulation by causing vasoconstriction and a decreased ability to sweat.
- The hyperthermic patient may therefore have impaired cooling ability.
- Conversely, vibration may also worsen the hypothermic patient's condition.

In addition, the flight environment poses specific problems:

- The outside temperature in the part of the atmosphere in which aircraft fly declines predictably with increasing altitude at a rate of approximately 2°C (3.6°F) every 1,000 ft.
- Temperature inside a pressurized cabin is controlled by the flight crew for the optimum comfort of the majority of passengers. This may not be suitable for your patient.

- The outside air which is used to pressurize the cabin is very cool, and therefore contains less water – the inside environment is therefore of very low humidity which can cause problems with respiratory and ophthalmic irritation and drying of bronchial secretions.

## ALTITUDE

### Composition and structure of the atmosphere

The atmosphere is a flexible, elastic envelope of mixed gases which surround the Earth. It extends up to about 500 miles, and is retained by the gravitational attraction of the planet. Conventionally, there are three layers (Figure 2.3) of which the most important, from a biological point of view is the troposphere. Most conventional passenger aircraft fly predominantly

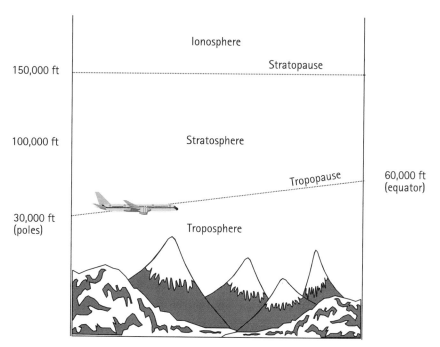

Fig. 2.3    The three layers of the atmosphere.

in the troposphere, and this layer is characterized by the presence of water vapour, a constant rate of decrease of temperature with increasing altitude, and the presence of large-scale vertical air currents (which mix the gases in to a fixed proportion at all altitudes).

*Air consists of matter:*
- It has the properties of mass and density (mass per unit volume).
- It can be compressed.
- The major components are oxygen (21%) and nitrogen (78%). For practical purposes, the remaining minority gases are ignored, since they play no part in normal respiratory physiology.
- The content of water vapour varies with location, altitude, and temperature. Warm air has a higher capacity to carry water vapour (a high humidity), compared with cold air.

## Atmospheric pressure and altitude

At sea level $1\,m^2$ column of air exerts a force of 10 t. This is called 1 atm, and can also be represented as 14.7 pounds per square inch (psi) or $1.03\,kg/cm^2$ (Figure 2.4). If the column is considered to be a stack of layers, it is easy to visualize how the bottom-most layer is compressed under the weight of all the molecules above it. In other words, the pressure at any point in the atmosphere is equal to the weight of all the molecules above it and therefore decreases with increasing altitude (Figure 2.5). More strictly, it is the force per unit area exerted by the weight of the atmosphere. One atmosphere is equal to 760 mmHg (also known as 760 torr). With the advent of *Systeme Internationale* units, pressure is now also measured in kilopascales (kPa), with 1 kPa equivalent to 7.6 mmHg, i.e. 1 atm (760 mmHg) = 100 kPa.

Since gases are compressible and more dense towards the surface, the relationship between pressure and altitude is not linear.

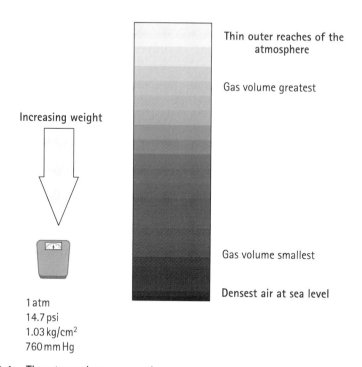

Thin outer reaches of the atmosphere

Gas volume greatest

Increasing weight

Gas volume smallest

Densest air at sea level

1 atm
14.7 psi
1.03 kg/cm²
760 mm Hg

Fig. 2.4    The atmosphere as a column.

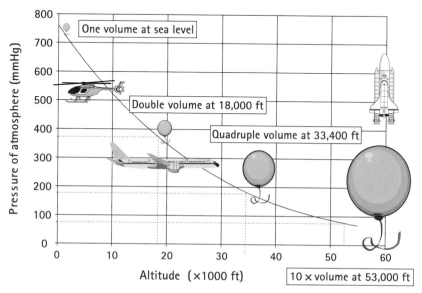

Fig. 2.5    The pressure–volume relationship with altitude.

In terms of pressure, half of the atmosphere occurs below 18,000 ft (i.e. ambient pressure is halved at 18,000 ft). An understanding of altitude physiology relies on an appreciation of the physical laws that dictate the behaviour of gases when exposed to reduced pressure. The most important is Boyle's law, which states that, at a constant temperature, the volume of a given mass of gas is inversely proportional to the pressure exerted upon it. It follows that, as density and pressure decrease with increasing altitude, the volume of gas will increase. Similarly, gas volumes will decrease on descent from altitude (Figure 2.6).

### The important physiological effects of altitude

On climbing through the atmosphere, although the relative composition of air remains constant, both pressure and density

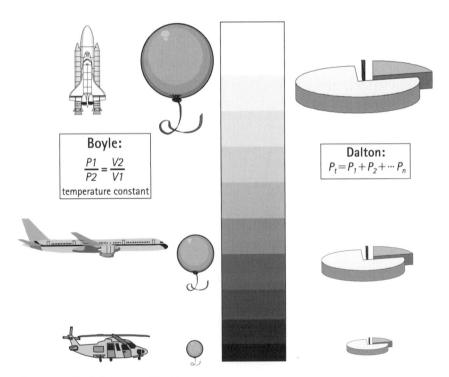

Fig. 2.6    Boyle's law and Dalton's law.

decline. Effectively this means that fewer oxygen molecules are available for physiological use and they are dispersed in a larger volume. The main concerns of altitude physiology are therefore hypoxia, i.e. oxygen deficiency sufficient to cause impairment of physiological function, and gas expansion within the body. Under normal circumstances, effects are minimal, but even healthy individuals are at danger in the event of an emergency rapid decompression of a pressurized cabin above 15,000 ft.

*Hypoxia*

The most relevant type of hypoxia in the flight environment is *hypobaric (hypoxic) hypoxia* which becomes apparent above 10,000 ft in healthy individuals. Without supplemental oxygen, blood oxygen saturation at sea level of 98% will decline to about 90% at 10,000 ft and 65% at 20,000 ft. Although hypoxic hypoxia is caused by an inadequate partial pressure of oxygen ($PO_2$) in inspired air, it is also experienced by those with a inadequate gas exchange at the alveolar-capillary membrane, ventilation/perfusion defect, or with an airway obstruction. Since these patients are hypoxic on the surface, they will clearly be at increased risk of hypoxic damage during flight.

Other forms of hypoxia will also exacerbate the complications of hypobaric hypoxia:

- *Hypaemic (anaemic) hypoxia* is caused by a reduction in the oxygen carrying capacity of the blood. This may be due to anaemia, hypovolemia, carbon monoxide poisoning, heavy smoking, or methaemaglobinemia (whether congenital or drug-induced).
- *Stagnant (circulatory) hypoxia* is oxygen deficiency due to reduction in tissue perfusion, such as in cardiogenic shock, or from venous pooling, arterial spasm, or occlusion of a blood vessel.

- *Histotoxic hypoxia* is the inability of the body tissues to utilize available oxygen, for instance with cyanide poisoning which uncouples oxidative phosphorylation.

### Signs and symptoms of hypoxia

The speed and order of appearance of signs and symptoms, and their severity, depend on the intensity of the hypoxic stimulus and the individual's demands on available oxygen. Influences on an individual's tolerance to hypoxia include:

- the altitude exposure,
- time at that altitude,
- previous acclimatization to altitude,
- extremes of ambient temperature,
- physical activity level,
- personal fitness,
- metabolic rate,
- diet and nutrition,
- emotions,
- fatigue,
- alcohol and some medications.

Transport in a pressurized cabin will reduce the potential for hypoxic complications but medical crew must be aware of predisposing medical conditions which can exacerbate hypoxia at altitude, i.e. any which interfere with gaseous exchange, oxygen carriage, or oxygen delivery.

Hypoxia is likely to be insidious in onset. The signs and symptoms can be predicted from the sensitivity of different tissue to a reduction in oxygen tension:

*Central nervous system (CNS)*   Neurons are extremely sensitive to hypoxia, especially in the higher areas of the brain (responsible for judgement, self-criticism, concentration, and mental tasks). Signs may begin when the alveolar $PO_2$ falls to 50–60 mmHg. At 45 mmHg, a hypoxically driven hyperventilation induces hypocapnia sufficient enough to cause cerebral vasoconstriction and decreased perfusion with further deterioration of mental abilities. Initial CNS signs and symptoms are usually those due to disinhibition:

- loquacity,
- euphoria,
- hyperactivity,
- restlessness.

Secondary signs and symptoms may include:

- limited attention span,
- impaired memory,
- deterioration of visual field and/or depth perception,
- depression,
- impaired judgement.

Progressive mental confusion, and unconsciousness will occur if exposure to hypoxia remains untreated. The arterial $PO_2$ at which unconsciousness occurs varies between 20 and 35 mmHg, depending on cerebral perfusion (i.e. on the balance of hypercapnia and hypoxia). Neuronal death begins when tissue $PO_2$ reaches 15 mmHg. The degree of brain damage to the individual, and whether or not it is reversible, will depend on the extent and location of areas exposed to sub-critical oxygen tensions.

*Respiratory system*    At about 5,000 ft, the initial respiratory response to hypoxia is an increase in the rate and tidal volume, i.e. the minute volume (MV). In effect, there is a balance between the increase in MV caused by the chemoreceptor response to hypoxia and the decrease in MV caused by hypoxic inhibition of the respiratory centres. Hyperventilation results in an overall reduction of carbon dioxide ($CO_2$) which causes a respiratory alkalosis and a shift of the oxygen dissociation curve to the left, increasing the affinity of haemoglobin for oxygen. The net effect is impaired oxygen delivery to the tissues.

*Cardiovascular system*    The cardiovascular system is relatively resistant to hypoxia. Heart rate will increase at altitude, rising to 15% greater than the sea level value at 15,000 ft and, although stroke volume (SV) remains unchanged, cardiac output (SV × heart rate (HR)) will increase accordingly. Vasodilation occurs in most areas, resulting in a fall in peripheral resistance. Physiological reflexes will try to maintain the systolic pressure, and pulse pressure will therefore widen. The resultant increase in cardiac activity will demand more oxygen and, if these needs are not met, the already hypoxic myocardium will eventually respond with a decrease heart rate, failure of contractility (reduction in SV) and dysrhythmias.

*Physiological stages of hypoxia*
   *Up to 10,000 ft*
- Oxygen saturation 90–98% in normal individuals.
- No awareness of symptoms and no noticeable impairment.

   *10,000–15,000 ft*
- Oxygen saturation 80–90% in normal individuals.
- Increase in respiratory rate, HR, and systolic blood pressure help to offset the decrease in oxygen carriage.
- Healthy individuals may remain asymptomatic.
- Some begin to experience nausea, dizziness, lethargy, headache, fatigue, and apprehension.
- After 15 min exposure: poor judgement, decreased efficiency, impaired co-ordination, and increased irritability may occur.

*15,000–20,000 ft*
- Oxygen saturation 70–80% in normal individuals.
- Physiological mechanisms can no longer compensate for the oxygen deficiency.
- Subjective symptoms of air hunger, headache, amnesia, decreased level of consciousness, and nausea occur.
- Impairment of visual acuity due to blurring or tunnel vision, and loss of colour clarity.
- Weakness, numbness, tingling and decreased sensation of touch and pain.
- Reaction time, cognitive function, short-term memory, speech and handwriting are greatly impaired.
- Behaviour may appear aggressive, belligerent, euphoric, overconfident or morose.
- Impaired muscular co-ordination makes delicate or fine movements impossible.
- Noticeable increase in respiratory rate, in the presence of central cyanosis.
- Muscular spasm and tetany may result from hypocapnia.
- Physical exertion at this stage will markedly exacerbate hypoxia and may rapidly lead to unconsciousness.

*Above 20,000 ft*
- Oxygen saturation 60–70% in normal individuals.
- Higher mental functions and neuromuscular control decline rapidly.
- Myoclonic jerking of the upper limbs and grand-mal-type seizures occur.
- Unconsciousness can occur with little or no warning.
- If hypoxia is not relieved immediately, irreversible cerebral damage will increase, and death will shortly follow.

*Treatment of hypoxia*

An understanding of the patient's clinical condition and of the physiological stresses of flight will help evaluate oxygen and pressure requirements for the journey. Recognition of signs and symptoms is a priority. Adequate monitoring of the patient during transport (e.g. electrocardiography (ECG), pulse oximetry and end-tidal capnography) is important. Supplemental oxygen remains the key to treatment:

*Supplemental oxygen*    The goal of oxygen therapy is to increase the arterial concentration of oxygen to meet the demands of tissue metabolism. Portable pulse oximetry can give medical crew valuable information about the response to oxygen therapy but its limitations must be understood. For instance, oximetry gives no information on oxygen carriage. Taken to the extreme, if a patient had only one red blood cell, and that cell was fully saturated, every time it passed the oximetry probe, the machine would read 100%. Clearly this patient is not carrying enough oxygen but this is not reflected in the saturation reading. The disadvantages of delivering 100% inspired oxygen concentration ($FIO_2$) throughout an entire long-haul journey include:

- respiratory tract irritation,
- substernal discomfort,
- ARDS-like phenomenon,
- delayed otic barotrauma,
- retrolental fibroplasia in premature neonates (if $PaO_2$ is allowed to rise too high),
- uneconomical,
- weight penalty incurred by carrying unnecessary oxygen cylinders.

For patients who are hypoxic at ground level, a recent blood gas result, preferably taken 'on air' is useful to help calculate altitude equivalence. Using Figure 2.7, the patient's arterial $PO_2$ can be compared against normal individuals to find the 'equivalent altitude'. This can be plotted on Figure 2.8 to give the $FIO_2$ needed to maintain an alveolar $PO_2$ of 100 mmHg. Constant reappraisal of the patient is essential and $FIO_2$ should be titrated to match clinical responses.

If, despite additional oxygen, evidence of hypoxia persists, consider depletion or malfunction of the onboard oxygen system, deterioration in the patient's condition, or that the patient cannot tolerate the change in barometric pressure.

*Gaseous expansion*
Several organs contain some form of gas. They may be filled with

- saturated air (in the paranasal sinuses and middle ear cavities),

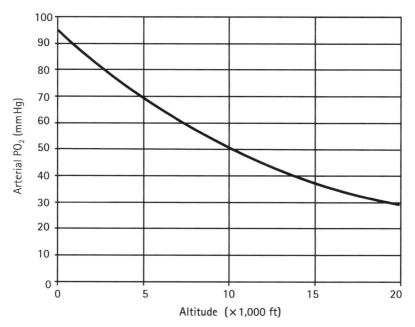

Fig. 2.7    Arterial $PO_2$ up to 20,000 ft, breathing air.

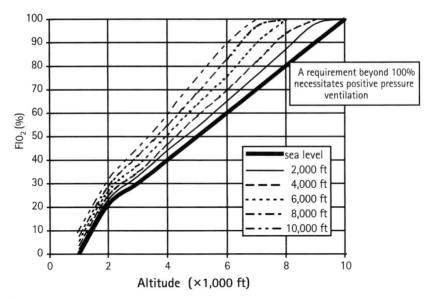

Fig. 2.8   The fractional concentration of oxygen required to maintain alveolar PO$_2$ of 100 mmHg.

- alveolar gas (saturated air enriched with carbon dioxide in the lungs),
- mixture of air and gases generated by digestive processes (in the gut).

These cavities communicate with the outside atmosphere with varying degrees of efficiency and the gas contained within them obeys Boyle's law, i.e. with decrease in ambient pressure, gas volume will expand (Figure 2.6). However, Boyle's law relates to dry gas. Gas in body cavities is saturated with water vapour at body temperature which exerts a constant vapour pressure of 47 mmHg. The net effect is that the greater the altitude, the greater the magnitude of gaseous expansion. If there is free venting between the gas-filled cavities and the outside atmosphere, expansion causes no difficulty or discomfort. Conversely, if the increase in volume cannot be vented, stretching of tissues may be painful. Ectopically located gas, such as in postoperative patients, or in those who have had gas or air introduced after an injury or as part of a diagnostic procedure is more problematic. Also, consider the effects of gas expansion on patients with ileus or gastric distension, and on items of medical equipment.

*Barotitis media (otic barotrauma)*   The middle ear is connected to the external atmosphere via the eustachian tube and is separated from the outer ear by the tympanic membrane. The eustachian tube usually functions as a one-way valve allowing gas to escape, but not return to the middle ear. Gas expands in the middle ear behind the tympanic membrane as altitude increases. It escapes through the eustachian tube every 500–1000 ft, or when there is a pressure differential of approximately 15 mmHg (felt as a 'popping'). On descent, the volume of gas in the middle ear contracts, creating a negative pressure and pulling the tympanic membrane inward. Under normal circumstances, the eustachian tube will not allow the passive movement of air into the middle ear but it can be opened by elevating the pressure in the nasopharynx by swallowing or the Frenzel manoeuvre (pinch the nose and blow). Inflammation of the mucosa (e.g. infection, allergy, or sinusitis) causes obstruction making equalization impossible. This is especially important in children with small diameter tubes which easily obstruct. If pressures are not equalized, symptoms may include 'fullness' in the ears, hearing loss as a result of decreased vibration of the drum, pain, tenderness, vertigo, nausea, perforation of the drum and bleeding. Treatment includes

- simple manoeuvres such as swallowing, valsalva, Frenzel, and moving the jaw,
- topical vasoconstrictor (decongestant) nasal spray may be beneficial,

- levelling off in the descent or an increase in altitude may be negotiated with the pilot so that symptoms are alleviated whilst waiting for vasoconstrictors to take effect,
- sleeping patients should be awoken 5 min before descent, so they can swallow more frequently,
- infants may be given a bottle during take-off and landing,
- slow descent from altitude will minimize the incidence and severity of symptoms,

*Barosinusitis (sinus barotrauma)*  Normally air can pass in and out of the sinus cavities freely and the only evidence of equilibration is a slight tickling sensation. If the mucous membrane lining of the sinuses is swollen, air may be trapped and will expand as altitude increases. The Frenzel manoeuvre is not effective in opening the blocked sinuses and symptoms soon develop. These may include severe pain in the cheek or forehead, lacrimation, and epistaxis. The treatment for barosinusitis is similar to the treatment of barotitis media, with the most effective being the use of a decongestant nasal spray and returning to a higher altitude.

*Barodontalgia*  Air trapped in dental fillings, decay, abscesses or crowns may result in a severe toothache, most commonly experienced during ascent. The only treatment, if it occurs in flight, is analgesia. Descent to lower altitude when pain is severe may be considered, if possible, and will certainly alleviate symptoms while waiting for analgesic medication to take effect.

*Abdominal distension*  The stomach and intestines normally contain up to 1 L of gas. Carbonated drinks, gas-producing foods, large meals, air swallowing and pre-existing gastro-intestinal infections may all increase the amount of gas in the gut. As gas expands on ascent, an individual may experience feelings of abdominal pressure, pain referred from diaphragmatic irritation, shortness of breath or hyperventilation from diaphragmatic splinting, nausea or even vomiting. Significant distension may result in venous pooling. In addition, tachycardia, hypotension, and syncope may result from a vasovagal response to severe pain. Prevention is the key:

- avoidance of gassy drinks and large meals prior to flight,
- especially those containing gas-producing foods such as dried peas and beans, pulses, cabbage, cauliflower, cucumber, turnip, sprouts, and high-roughage foods such as celery and bran,
- loose non-restrictive clothing may be of benefit,
- sufferers should not be modest at venting expanding gas to relieve discomfort,
- patients with a bowel obstruction, ileus, or recent abdominal surgery must have a patent free-draining NG tube in place prior to transport.

*The respiratory system*   The lungs freely communicate with the outside atmosphere and, except in the rare circumstance of emergency rapid decompression, no problem will be encountered with pressure equalization. However, expansion of pleural gas in an inadequately vented pneumothorax will cause further collapse of pulmonary tissue. Patients can be safely transported once a chest tube is in place but careful monitoring for evidence of hypoxia or occlusion of the chest tube throughout the journey is essential. Artificially ventilated patients must be closely monitored for the development of a tension pneumothorax.

## Cabin pressurization

An ideal aircraft cabin might be expected to have an internal pressure set to 1 atm (760 mmHg), but the penalties (weight of the cabin and pressurization equipment, the power requirements, and the risks of large pressure differentials across the cabin wall) would be insurmountable. A compromise cabin pressure between 6,000 and 8,000 ft allows the occupants to breathe air in comfort, and with minimal risk of explosive decompression due to structural failure. Pressurization is made possible by the indrawing of air from the outside. It is compressed by engine-driven compressors and delivered to the cabin where the pressure is maintained by controlling flow out of the aircraft.

### Rapid decompression

Rapid decompression is an unusual event in civilian aircraft, but may occur if the cabin wall is breached, or with malfunction of the pressure control system. Pressure initially falls rapidly, and then more slowly as internal pressure equilibrates with the lower-ambient pressure outside. The injurious effects on the aircraft occupants are:

- *Air blast.* Until air pressures equilibrate, the velocity of air flow around the defect will be great. Dust, debris and loose articles will be sucked by the wind flow.
- *Cold.* The rapid expansion of air as it equilibrates to a lower pressure reduces its temperature. The eventual cabin temperature will depend on the size of the defect, the outside air temperature, and the aircraft's altitude and speed.
- *Misting.* Cold air holds less water than warm air. Sudden cooling of air as it expands causes misting as water vapour condenses out of the cooling air mass.
- *Gaseous expansion.* If emergency decompression occurs while the glottis is closed, the lungs may suffer barotrauma as trapped gas expands rapidly. This may result in simple or tension pneumothorax.

- *Decompression sickness (DCS).* The incidence of DCS is insignificant below 30,000 ft and is virtually unheard of in civilian aircraft. However, its occurrence is more likely in occupants who are ill, have been recently injured, or who are overweight.
- *Hypoxia.* Hypoxic effects may be rapid in onset with catastrophic hypoxaemia occurring within seconds if rapid decompression equilibrates above 30,000 ft. Above this altitude, alveolar $PO_2$ is lower than venous $PO_2$ with the result that oxygen passes out of the blood into the lungs and is expired with each breath. Although unconsciousness may occur within half a minute, mental impairment can occur even quicker, and sensible, reasoned actions may become impossible.

## FATIGUE AND JET LAG DURING LONG-HAUL FLIGHTS

### Circadian rhythms

Human circadian rhythms exert a pattern of sleep and wakefulness that is closely related to the 24 h day–night cycle. Almost all homeostatic functions oscillate in this manner, and the overall pattern of circadian rhythmicity can be measured by body temperature, plasma cortisol release, and melatonin. The most important influence on circadian rhythms are

- daily alternation between light and dark,
- temperature,
- activity,
- artificial or social synchronizers called *zeitgebers* (time-givers), such as clocks, meal-times, and radio/TV programmes.

The ability to sleep varies with the phase of the temperature cycle but the oscillator is slow to change and it is difficult to adjust sleep patterns rapidly after a time zone change (jet lag). Alterations in circadian rhythms reduce effectiveness and impair psychomotor performance, hence adequate and good quality sleep is essential.

### Transmeridian (east–west) flights

Jet lag occurs when travel across time zones takes the human body rapidly into another phase of the 24 h day–night cycle at a speed which exceeds the ability of synchronizers to entrain physiological rhythms. The subsequent desynchronization leads to

- excessive tiredness – over and above the fatigue caused by the flight,
- generalized discomfort and malaise,
- sleep disturbance,
- loss of appetite,
- disruptions of feeding pattern and bowel habit,
- sub-optimal levels of performance at important times of the day.

There is great individual variation in the effects of jet lag and there are many suggestions on its management:

- Sleeping on the aircraft (not practicable for single medical crew escorting patients, but may be possible during the staging flight).
- Avoidance of heavy meals and alcohol.
- Planning of a suitable work schedule.
- Mild hypnotics (e.g. temazepam), help to ensure adequate rest but have no direct influence on the rate at which re-entrainment occurs.

- Melatonin, taken prior to sleep, appears to advance the circadian cycle and encourages sleep, possibly by lowering body temperature.

Sleep after transmeridian flights is influenced by the timing of the flight and the direction of travel. Westward flights, say with a sleep period delay of 5 h, enable individuals to fall asleep quickly and sleep more soundly in the first rest period after the flight. The only detrimental effect is likely to be less restful sleep during the latter part of the night as one tries to extend sleep toward the local time of rising.

If sleep can be avoided during an eastbound flight (i.e. if the 'natural' rest period is ignored), once the immediate effect of sleep loss is overcome, the first sleep after the journey will be of good quality. Paradoxically, though, quality of sleep is likely to deteriorate over the next few days and adaptation may take longer.

## North–south long-haul flights

Many north–south flights are scheduled overnight. Since few or no time zones are crossed, the predominant problem is one of sleep deprivation. To some extent, fatigue can be prevented by adequate sleep prior to departure. Napping may also appear to help tiredness, but tests show that alertness and performance deteriorate despite most individuals subjectively feeling less tired after the nap.

Some aspects of flight common to all long-distance journeys are also likely to worsen fatigue:

- the mild hypoxia experienced at altitude,
- low humidity,
- extremes of temperature,
- vibration,
- noise,

- boredom,
- relative inactivity.

### Planning medical crew duty times

The combination of irregular work patterns and sleep disturbance greatly impairs alertness and performance. Performance during long shifts is influenced by four main factors:

- time elapsed since start of duty,
- time of day,
- adaptation to local time zone,
- time since last sleep.

For an individual who is fully rested at the start of a duty period performance improves on task over the first 5 h. It then tends to drop precipitously and falls to a plateau at about 16 h of time-on-task.

A time zone-adapted individual (entrained in normal circadian rhythms) will perform best in the afternoon. Performance then declines until it reaches a trough at about 05:00 in the morning (i.e. the nadir of the circadian cycle). Those who organize aeromedical schedules should avoid situations which might lead to the superimposition of the low plateau of time-on-task and the circadian nadir. Performance under these circumstances is significantly worse than at either of the low points independently. The situation is further compounded by insufficient or poor quality rest prior to the start of duty, and when time zones are crossed. The consequences for patient care are obvious.

### Clinical problems of long–haul travel

The consequences of the journey to the patient (not just the flight, but also the ground transfers at either end), must be considered. Least at risk will be those who are sedated and being transferred on stretchers. Paradoxically, it is usually the ambulant patient who suffers most. Patients are often stressed before they arrive at the busy and chaotic environment of the airport. This is worsened as they pass through the tedious but essential formalities necessary before boarding. Patients have the added anxieties of their illness; they may also be leaving relatives behind, and may seem disproportionately worried about seemingly less-important matters, such as ensuring that baggage has been checked in, and so on. All these apprehensions may cause or worsen sleep disturbance and feelings of well-being.

Give careful thought to timings of drugs, meals and treatments. In particular, some drugs are time-dependent (such as insulin, thyroxine, and the progestin *minipill*). The simplest answer is to maintain the patient on the local standard time of the point of departure throughout the journey. Drugs, treatments, and meals should continue to be given at the expected times, and the patient's watch should not be changed to the destination time zone. It must be clearly documented in the patient's transfer record that drugs and treatments were given at local times and this information must be passed on to the handover team at the destination hospital.

## FURTHER READING

Anton DJ (1988) Crash dynamics and restraint systems. In: Ernsting J, King PF (eds) Aviation Medicine (2nd edn). Butterworth: London.

Benson AJ (1988) Motion sickness. In: Ernsting J, King PF (eds) Aviation Medicine (2nd edn). Butterworth: London.

Blumen IJ (1995) Altitude physiology and the stresses of flight. Air Med J 14(2): 87–99.

Ernsting J, Sharp GR, Harding RM (1988) Hypoxia and hyperventilation. In: Ernsting J, King PF (eds) Aviation Medicine (2nd edn). Butterworth: London.

Ernsting J, Sharp GR, Macmillan AJF (1988) Prevention of hypoxia below 40,000 feet. In: Ernsting J, King PF (eds) Aviation Medicine (2nd edn). Butterworth: London.

Glaister DH (1988) The effects of long duration acceleration. In: Ernsting J, King PF (eds) Aviation Medicine (2nd edn). Butterworth: London.

Harding RM, Mills FJ (1993) Acceleration. In: Harding RM, Mills FJ (eds) Aviation Medicine (3rd edn). BMJ: London.

Harding RM, Mills FJ (1993) Problems of altitude. In: Harding RM, Mills FJ (eds) Aviation Medicine (3rd edn). BMJ: London.

Martin TC (1995) Adverse effects of rotating schedules on the circadian rhythms of air medical crews. Air Med J 14(2): 83–86.

Martin TE, Rodenberg HD (1996) Aeromedical Transportation: A Clinical Guide. Avebury: Aldershot.

McFarland RA (1974) Influence of changing time zones on aircrew and passengers. Aerospace Med 45: 648–658.

Pascoe PA (1992) Jet lag. In: Dawood R (ed.) Travellers' Health (3rd edn). Oxford University Press: Oxford.

Rood GM (1988) Noise and communication. In: Ernsting J, King PF (eds) Aviation Medicine (2nd edn). Butterworth: London.

Stott JRR (1988) Vibration. In: Ernsting J, King PF (eds) Aviation Medicine (2nd edn). Butterworth: London.

# 3

# Stabilization prior to transportation

The process of transferring a patient from the scene of an accident or during an interhospital transfer causes additional physiological stresses to the already compromised patient. In addition, it may be difficult to perform certain procedures while in transit. This is particularly true in small helicopter air ambulances where space may be at a premium and it may be difficult to reach parts of the patient. Other environments for patient transfer create challenges, e.g. the need for privacy when a patient is being transferred aboard a commercial passenger aeroplane. It is therefore essential that the patient is optimally prepared for the journey. The following considerations need to be addressed:

- The urgency with which the patient must reach the destination.
- The mode of transportation.
- The interventions which will benefit the patient if done before transfer.
- The investigations which will benefit the patient if done before transfer.

- Procedures which may be necessary during transfer.
- Special consideration of the environment in which the patient will be placed during transfer.
- The experience of the escort undertaking the transfer.

The primary transfer and interhospital transfer may have very different priorities. Although the principles are the same for both, they will be considered separately for reasons of clarity. In both cases, the structured approach to the problem is, as usual, based on A, B, C – assessment and management of the airway followed by breathing and then the circulation.

## PRIMARY TRANSFER – SCOOP AND RUN, OR STAY AND PLAY?

The diversity of the prehospital environment poses many problems and the decision when to move is often widely debated. The aim of any primary transfer is to deliver the patient as soon as possible to hospital, with the minimum of deterioration and preferably some improvement in clinical condition. The amount of treatment provided on scene and the degree of stabilization that is achieved before moving the patient will depend on the circumstances. Generally, before providing any specific treatment or intervention to a critically ill patient which will delay transfer to definitive care, the rescuer must be satisfied that the delay in transfer is justified. The decision when to move will depend on

- the condition of the patient,
- the distance (in time) from the receiving unit,
- the training and number of personnel available,
- the equipment available.

### The condition of the patient

This should follow an 'ABC' approach, i.e. airway compromise is more urgent than a breathing problem. If the airway and breathing cannot be stabilized on scene, immediate transportation is essential. The spine should be immobilized if there is any sugestion of damage, for instance

- pain in the neck or back of a conscious patient,
- neurological symptoms or signs suggestive of a cord injury in any patient,
- significant injury above the clavicles in an unconscious patient,
- suggestive mechanism of injury in an unconscious patient.

Conversely, providing entrapment is not an issue, the circulation is often best addressed in transit. Running intravenous (IV) fluids through a giving set and finding a suitable vein may easily be performed whilst the ambulance is travelling. If necessary the vehicle can be stopped briefly at the roadside once everything is prepared for cannulation. It may be necessary to secure IV access before leaving the scene if air transportation is being used to cover a long distance.

## The distance (in time) from the receiving unit

This must also be considered when deciding whether to provide on-scene treatment or not. The decision to transfer will depend on the urgency of the intervention required, but sometimes it is better to 'scoop and run' if the distance is short, particularly in conditions where better outcome is known to be related to short on-scene and transfer times.

The *mode* of transportation in primary transfer will usually be road ambulance but may be a helicopter – which needs extra considerations whilst 'packaging' the patient. Selection of transport mode depends on

- urgency of the transfer,
- distance to appropriate receiving unit,

- availability,
- logistics and terrain – e.g. weather, time of day, and availability of helicopter landing sites at the scene and at the receiving unit.

In addition special modifications to the method of transport may be necessary:

- Spinal injury may require a slow police escort for a smooth journey.
- Low-flying requirements may be necessary in certain clinical circumstances, such as when gaseous expansion at altitude can exacerbate a pneumothorax (especially if no chest drain has been inserted on-scene), and also for patients with decompression sickness.

### The training and number of personnel available

This can vary enormously outside hospital. If a British Association of Immediate Care Schemes (BASICS) or HEMS doctor is present, it may be possible for more advanced procedures to be provided at an earlier stage (e.g. rapid sequence induction anaesthesia for head injury). Specialized procedures may save lives, but increase the on-scene time considerably. Prehospital time must be minimized when rescuers have minimal skills.

### The equipment available

This will clearly influence the decision on what can be achieved prior to transport even if skilled personnel are present.

## SECONDARY TRANSFER – INTERHOSPITAL AND INTRAHOSPITAL TRANSFERS

Once hospital has been reached, even if it is not the final destination, more extensive resources are available in terms of expertise, equipment, communications, and investigations. The patient's condition should be stabilized and optimized, including any investigations which may help to decide on the need for secondary transfer. These should not cause undue delay. The primary survey and initial resuscitation must be completed before secondary transfer, unless an aspect of resuscitation cannot be provided without transfer (such as laparotomy for uncontrolled haemorrhage) in which case the transfer essentially becomes part of the resuscitation.

There are a number of areas that must be addressed:

### Communication

This must include direct liaison between the referring and receiving clinicians. Essential details are

- the clinical state of the patient,
- whether the patient is fit to transfer (is there a significant risk of deterioration?),
- treatment received so far,
- treatment required (the reason for the transfer),
- which hospital/department will conduct the transfer and how,
- any treatment or investigations required by the receiving unit before transfer.

Although it is essential the two units work together, the clinical responsibility remains with the referring clinician until the patient is taken over by the receiving unit staff, either by their retrieval team or on arrival at their facility.

### ABC checklist

Following the decision to transfer, the patient must be methodically assessed using an 'airway, breathing, and circulation' checklist and suitable precautions taken for any foreseeable mishaps or deterioration that might occur during the transfer. The following points must be addressed.

### Airway

- Is the airway patent?
- Is the airway secure, bearing in mind patient movement? Elective endotracheal intubation should be undertaken if there is any doubt that the airway may become compromised in transit. The natural history of some airway problems such as respiratory burns is to worsen with time. In addition, any patient who may not be able to protect his own airway, such as those with a diminished conscious level (particularly in those with severe head injury, in whom optimal oxygenation may be life-saving) should be intubated with a cuffed endotracheal tube. Ideally, a chest X-ray should confirm tube position before transfer.

### Cervical spine

- Where indicated, ensure the spine is adequately immobilized. Although patients with spinal injuries may be conveniently nursed in transit using a vacuum mattress, a firm stretcher should be placed underneath for lifting.

### Breathing

- Is the breathing stabilized?
- In the case of possible chest injury or post-intubation, a chest X-ray should be performed before transfer.
- If there is any doubt that the patient's breathing may become compromised during the journey, he should be electively ventilated. This includes patients with injuries such as a significant flail chest and any other condition where oxygenation or ventilation may be impaired.

- Any pneumothorax should be assessed and, particularly if air transportation is to be used, a chest drain inserted prior to transfer and attached to a valved drainage bag or Heimlich valve.
- In ventilated patients or those with breathing difficulties, the arterial blood gases should be checked before leaving.

### Circulation

- Access to the circulation should be secured by a minimum of two peripheral wide bore IV cannulae. More secure access such as a central venous line may also be indicated and this should be sutured in place.
- External haemorrhage should be controlled.
- Shock should be treated with appropriate IV fluids. If cardiogenic shock is a contributory factor, inotropic support should be initiated and a central venous pressure (CVP) line is required for added monitoring.
- Fractures should be immobilized to minimize pain and ongoing blood loss.
- A urinary catheter should be inserted to monitor end-organ perfusion.
- Blood should be drawn for full blood count and cross matched if necessary. If taken during the journey, it should be transported in a box designed for the purpose to prevent deterioration.

### Other procedures/investigations

- Unless contraindicated, a nasogastric or orogastric tube should be inserted in any critically ill patient prior to transfer and left to drain freely into a bag. It should also be aspirated frequently.
- The urea, electrolytes and blood glucose should be measured as a baseline. Where it is likely that they may be

seriously disturbed, it is essential to wait for the result before initiating the transfer.

- Adequate analgesia should be given prior to moving the patient.
- Under certain circumstances, anti-emetics may be required to prevent motion sickness.
- The patient must be equipped for the environment he is going to face. If he is already cold or if it is likely that he will be exposed to cold for any length of time (in an ambulance, between hospital buildings or on an airport runway), suitable blankets must be prepared. Occasionally umbrellas or plastic sheeting may also be needed to protect from rain or snow.
- Any other requirements of the environment; e.g. if the transfer is by commercial passenger aeroplane, has suitable attention been give to personal requirements and privacy?

*Monitoring equipment*
It is important to monitor the patient as adequately as in a hospital bed. A sick patient requires a minimum of

- ECG,
- pulse oximetry,
- non-invasive BP.

It may be possible to use monitoring equipment provided by the ambulance whilst in transit, but portable machinery will also be necessary for the transfer to and from the vehicle.

In addition, the following may be required:

- End tidal-$CO_2$.
- Invasive monitoring for BP and CVP. These require sophisticated monitors that are not routinely available in

transportation vehicles. The patient needs to be attached to these monitors before leaving the referring department.

- IV fluids will require infusion pumps.

*Final checklist*
- Is the airway secure?
- Is the patient protected from aspiration?
- Is the spine adequately immobilized (where necessary)?
- Is the breathing adequate and are the blood gases satisfactory?
- Has shock been treated?
- Does the patient have adequate IV access?
- Is a urinary catheter in place (where indicated)?
- Have all special environmental considerations been taken into account?
- Is appropriate monitoring in place including infusion pumps?

## FURTHER READING

American College of Surgeons (1997) Advanced Trauma Life Support for Doctors (6th edn). ACS: Chicago.

Langford SA (1991) Preparation of Patients for Transport. Monograph series number 2. Royal Flying Doctor Service: Hurstville.

Martin TE, Rodenberg HD (1996) Aeromedical Transportation: A Clinical Guide. Avebury: Aldershot.

Morton NS, Murray MP, Wallace PGM (1997) Stabilization and Transport of the Critically Ill. Churchill Livingstone: London.

# 4

# Logistics of ground transportation

## INTRODUCTION

There are many reasons to transport patients:

- Primary transfer from the scene of an accident or emergency.
- Emergency interhospital transfers (usually inter-ITU or other critical care facility).
- Emergency intrahospital transfers (e.g. from a helipad to A&E, or between hospital buildings).
- Non-urgent interhospital transfers.
- Transport of patients to outpatient appointments.
- Routine admissions.
- Taking some patients home from hospital, or to and from a day-centre.

Individual patient requirements vary considerably. The needs of an active 60-year old coming for an outpatient visit will be quite different to those of a critically ill premature baby being transferred for emergency surgery in a transport incubator system. It is important to ensure that the ambulance service understands exactly what the nature of the transfer is to be. In exceptional circumstances, trains, buses, and other types of vehicles may be used for patient transportation.

## AMBULANCE SERVICES

The UK Ambulance Service comprises 66 individual services which generally correspond with county and metropolitan boundaries:

- 43 in England,
- 8 in Scotland,
- 9 in Wales,
- 4 in Northern Ireland,
- 1 in Jersey,
- 1 in Guernsey.

Individual services therefore vary greatly in size, depending on the area they serve. They are responsible for providing accident and emergency and patient transport services for the population within their catchment areas, and must meet standards set by the Department of Health:

- 100% of all emergency call must be answered (and a vehicle dispatched) within 3 min,
- 50% of all emergency calls must have an ambulance in attendance within 8 min,
- 95% of all calls must have an ambulance in attendance within 19 min.

In addition to the 999 response, the accident and emergency service caters for general practitioners (GPs) urgent admissions and also the transfers of patients who require high-dependency care. The patient transport service meets the transport needs of outpatients and other non-urgent transfers, as well as providing extra vehicles for major incidents.

The main type of ground vehicle used for transporting patients is the road ambulance. Ambulances come in various shapes and sizes depending on the purpose for which they are used:

- The familiar frontline paramedic emergency vehicle (Figure 4.1).
- Ambulance minibus for outpatient transport (Figure 4.2).
- Four-wheel drive vehicles for rough terrain (Figure 4.3).
- Special purpose vehicles, such as for neonatal or intensive care transfers (Figure 4.4).
- Conventional cars as rapid response vehicles and for BASICS doctors (Figure 4.5).

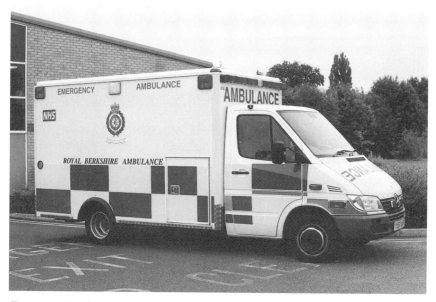

Fig. 4.1 The frontline paramedic emergency vehicle.

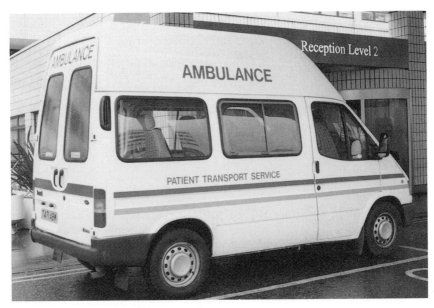

Fig. 4.2    Ambulance patient transport service minibus.

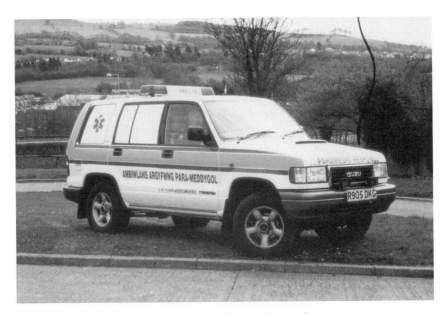

Fig. 4.3    Four-wheel drive ambulance for rough terrain.

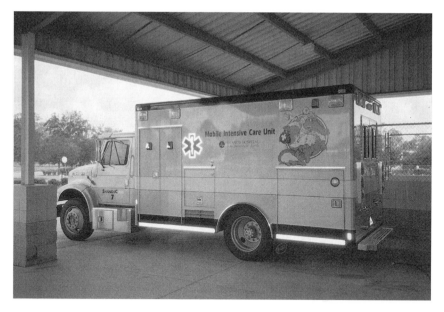

Fig. 4.4    Special purpose vehicle for neonatal or intensive care transfers.

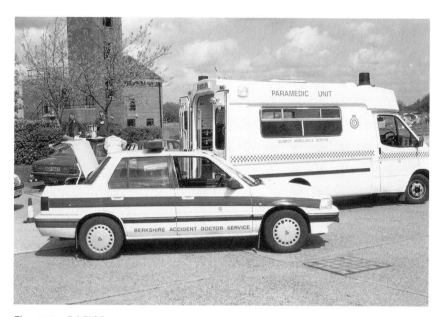

Fig. 4.5    BASICS car.

## RETRIEVAL TEAMS

When a hospital offers a retrieval service for critically ill patients, there must be close liaison with the local ambulance service. This type of transfer will arise frequently and often at short notice. There will be no time for confusion or indecision. Logistic considerations that should be taken into account when setting up such a service include:

- How will the retrieval team reach the referring hospital?
- Will a dedicated ambulance be allocated to such a service?
- If not, will the ambulance come from the referring hospital's ambulance service or will the team be transported to the referring hospital using the ambulance which will bring them (and the patient) back?
- What equipment will be provided by the ambulance service and what by the hospital?
- Is the hospital equipment compatible with the vehicle(s) to be used, in terms of electrical voltage and fittings?
- If not, what adaptations need to be made to the equipment and/or vehicles?
- What role will the paramedics/ambulance technicians play, and what will be the composition and training of the hospital team?
- And finally, from where will funding be obtained?

When a call is received to collect a patient, this planning and organization should be put into practice and, hopefully, most contingencies will have been considered. Such a system is clearly the most desirable method of moving critically ill patients and will have the additional advantages of dedicated equipment, staff, and sometimes a vehicle. Similar planning is required for those hospitals that offer a 'trauma team' from the emergency department to assist paramedics at major accidents.

## EMERGENCY INTERHOSPITAL TRANSFERS

### Preparation

Where a retrieval service is not in place or appropriate, a number of factors have to be addressed on each occasion that a patient is to be transferred. Firstly, the ambulance service need to know certain information regarding the proposed transfer. This includes the following points.

### Who/what is to be transported?

For instance, not all vehicles have the fittings required for a transport incubator, and an extraordinarily heavy patient may require extra attendants to lift him.

### What is the patient's condition?

Although the hospital staff may be responsible for the medical care, some aspects are still important to the ambulance service. They particularly need to know if the patient is infectious (the vehicle will be out of action for longer because of the need for special cleaning) or if the patient has a psychiatric problem (e.g. are they going to try to leap out of the moving vehicle).

### Where is the patient's final destination?

If it is a long distance, they may need to call in staff early for a shift, and the driver needs to be certain of the route. If the routing is unclear, ambulance control will arrange for the ambulance crew to speak to the destination ambulance control once they are in the area, so that an escort for the vehicle can be arranged.

### When will the journey take place?

To ensure vehicle availability, the ambulance service need as much notice as possible of the day and approximate time. Confirmation of the exact time the patient is expected to be ready is required nearer the time, so that they can continue with their normal work until the transfer is about to take place.

### Who is accompanying the patient?

There must be enough room in the ambulance for everyone. Under certain circumstances, e.g. during a neonatal transfer where the mother is also to travel, it may even be that two ambulances are required – especially if the mother has recently delivered or is unwell.

### Is a police escort required?

The police can ensure the ambulance has a clear fast run to the destination by warning other drivers of its presence and by blocking junctions and clearing traffic. However this kind of driving is not without danger to the public, all those travelling in the ambulance, and to the police outriders themselves. A police escort should only be undertaken if the risk to the patient of the transfer is very considerable. Particular points to consider when deciding if a police escort is appropriate are as follows:

- What will be the danger to the patient if the transfer takes longer than the minimum amount of time?
- The time of day (will it be rush hour?).
- The weather (snow, ice, fog, and driving rain).

Remember that the police may also supply a slow escort to ensure a constant, smooth journey for patients with conditions such as spinal injury.

### Are the accompanying staff to be returned to their point of origin?

If it is only a short journey the medical team may be required to make their own way back to the hospital, but on long journeys it is usual for the ambulance crew to wait while the patient is handed over to the receiving unit and then transport the staff and equipment back to their own unit.

There are also a number of issues which need to be discussed directly with the ambulance crew when they arrive to collect the patient.

*Whose equipment is to be used?*

Usually it is a mixture of both – e.g. bringing a second defibrillator when the ambulance already has one will use up unnecessary space. It is usual to use the oxygen supplied in the vehicle. Ensure that, if the ambulance equipment is to be used, that it is appropriate for the patient – e.g. some vehicles carry semi-automatic defibrillators which are unsuitable for use in children. Never assume that the paramedics have certain drugs or equipment. If the plan is to rely on their supply, check that each item is, in fact, available and suitable.

*What oxygen supply will be taken?*

Be sure that you know how to calculate the oxygen requirements for the needs of the patient and do so, then have double the anticipated volume available for the journey. For example, for an E-size cylinder (commonly used portable size),

$$\text{Minutes of oxygen available} = \text{pressure (in psi)} \times 0.3 \text{ /flow/L/min.}$$

*Final checks before departure*

- Check that the driver knows the way to the receiving hospital.
- Check the fittings are appropriate for the equipment accompanying the patient.
- Check that the ambulance battery voltage is compatible with any electrical equipment to be brought and that connectors fit satisfactorily. If they do not, ensure that enough battery power is available for the whole journey and some extra battery time is allowed for emergencies.

- Tell the paramedic/emergency medical technician (EMT) what you anticipate his role to be. If he is needed to participate in clinical care, he should be aware of what he is expected to do.

## ROUTINE PATIENT TRANSPORT SYSTEM

This type of transportation rarely involves doctors or nurses in its execution but if requesting an ambulance for a non-urgent patient (e.g. to attend outpatients) there are some points that should be observed:

- To avoid unavailability, usually a minimum booking time is required, often 48 h in advance. Failure to reserve an ambulance early may mean that the patient has to be transported using an emergency vehicle – an expensive resource – or, indeed, may not be able to travel.
- Ambulance control needs to know if the patient is able to walk, is in a chair or must be transported on a stretcher.
- They need to know about infection precautions, psychiatric, or extraordinary weight requirements (as above).
- They need to know if the patient will be accompanied.

## MAJOR INCIDENTS

Extraordinary logistics come into play when a major incident occurs (Figure 4.6). Indeed one definition of such an occurrence for the health service is when 'there are, or likely to be so many casualties that special arrangements are necessary to deal with them'. Major incident planning is beyond the scope of this text and plans vary from area to area. However, it is worthy of

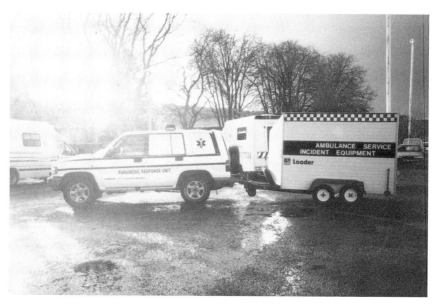

Fig. 4.6   Ambulance control major incident vehicle.

mention the following information:

- Non-emergency vehicles (such as outpatients transport) may be re-deployed early in the incident to assist with injured patients who do not require the facilities of an emergency vehicle.
- Other modes of transportation may be used in such circumstances such as specially converted coaches (Figure 4.7). Trains may be particularly useful in transporting large numbers of casualties and have been used in both military and civilian disasters for over a hundred years (Figure 4.8). Dedicated rescue trains may be particularly useful in certain types of accident such as railway tunnel accidents. The only civilian train in the UK designed for such an eventuality is the Severn tunnel rescue train, capable of carrying 10 casualties. In contrast, Germany, where there are many long railway tunnels, has six tunnel-rescue trains, comprehensively equipped in terms

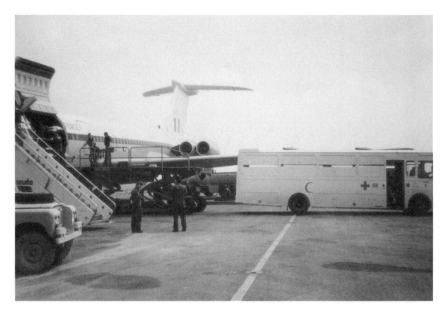

Fig. 4.7    Coach used to evacuate casualties after a major disaster.

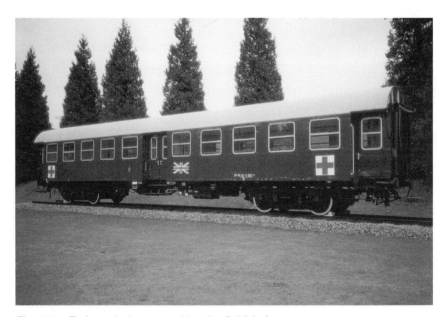

Fig. 4.8    Train ambulance used by the British Army.

of both medical and rescue equipment and each capable of carrying 60 casualties. Trains may also be useful in secondary transfer when spreading the load between hospitals following a major incident.

## FURTHER READING

Beaulieu P, Vilain L (1997) Primary transport. In: Morton NS et al. (eds) Stabilization and Transport of the Critically Ill. Churchill Livingstone: London.

Robertson B (1994) Potential of trains in disaster situations. Disaster Manag. 6(2): 91–95.

# 5

# Logistics of intrahospital transfers

Safe intrahospital transfer of patients requires meticulous, detailed organization, and the implementation of a formulated plan. The fundamental principle of a high-quality intrahospital transfer is that the level of care prior to transfer must be maintained throughout the transfer until the patient arrives at the final destination.

The decision to transfer a patient for an investigation or specialized care to another part of the hospital may appear to be a purely medical one at first. However, it is in almost all cases a team effort, as it involves several professional groups. Other professional groups may wish to reschedule their interventions or therapy, e.g. the physiotherapist may wish to undertake physiotherapy prior to the patient's transfer for maximum effect. The patient's and relative's wishes must also be considered. Pre-planning may be facilitated by answering the following 10 questions:

- Is the transfer absolutely necessary?
- What are the benefits of transferring the patient?
- What are the risks of transfer?

- Where is the transfer to and what is the most reliable and expeditious route?
- When should the transfer occur?
- Which staff should be undertaking the transfer?
- Which preparations of the patient are necessary, and are there any additional special precautions?
- What equipment is required for the transfer?
- Is the equipment available and ready to use?
- What else needs to be taken on the transfer (e.g. transfer documentation, case notes, X-rays, and investigation request forms)?

Close liaison and ongoing communication with the receiving department are essential. The transfer team should be given a time window of 'when to be there', rather than a fixed time. Frequently there will be unforeseeable last minute problems to be sorted out. Equally the transfer team should keep the receiving team informed about any changes in plan, such as cancellation when there is no longer an indication for the transfer, or postponement due to sudden deterioration of the patient. If transport time is long, immediately prior to setting off the team should pass on an estimated time of arrival. Checklists for the transfer equipment and patient preparation are useful (Figures 5.1–5.4). Ideally they are incorporated into the transfer documentation and checked off by two people.

When returning to the point of origin, the timing of the return journey and any special requirements should be communicated. Often additional staff are required to set up the bed space, or to help transfer the patient back into a bed. Senior medical staff should ideally re-assess the patient's condition and debrief the transfer team.

Each journey ends with the completion of transfer documentation and, if required, critical incident reporting. These are essential for audit, further training, and quality assurance.

| Is your equipment ready for transfer? | Yes | Comments |
|---|---|---|
| Transfer trolley available? | | |
| Cylinder oxygen supplies full and functional? | | |
| Syringe drivers and infusion pumps fully charged? | | |
| Transfer backpack fully equipped with ABC equipment? | | |
| Check laryngoscope and carry spare batteries? | | |
| Check patient's treatment chart? | | |
| Appropriate drugs and infusions prepared? | | |
| Resuscitation drugs available? | | |
| Anaesthetic drugs available? | | |
| Refrigerator drugs still usable? | | |
| Transport ventilator with filter functional? | | |
| Multi-modality monitor fully charged and functional? | | |
| Transducer leads, oximeter finger probe and BP cuff available? | | |
| End-tidal $CO_2$ probe available? | | |
| Suction unit functional? | | |
| Defibrillator operational? | | |
| Warming blanket needed? | | |
| Transfer documentation form commenced? | | |
| Anything else we might need or anything missing? | | |

Fig. 5.1   Checklist for equipment.

| Is the team ready for transfer? | Yes | Comments |
|---|---|---|
| Does the transfer team have the appropriate expertise? | | |
| Do they have enough knowledge of the location and the case? | | |
| Is the patient stable? (pre-transfer vital signs and arterial blood gases if appropriate) | | |
| Are case notes, X-ray films, laboratory results and request forms collected? | | |
| Has the receiving department been informed about imminent departure and estimated time of arrival? | | |
| Has the porter been informed? | | |

Fig. 5.2   Checklist for team preparation.

| Is the patient ready for transfer? | Yes | Comments |
|---|---|---|
| Is the patient informed about the planned transfer? | | |
| Are the relatives informed and aware of the Transfer? | | |
| Have drugs, pumps and lines been rationalized and secured? | | |
| Are intubation and ventilation required? | | |
| Are sedation, analgesia and neuromuscular block adequate? | | |
| Is the airway secure? | | |
| Is the patient breathing appropriately? | | |
| Are partial pressure of $O_2$ and $CO_2$ ($PO_2$ and $PCO_2$) appropriate? | | |
| Are chest drains working appropriately? | | |
| Any evidence of overt or occult bleeding? | | |
| Is intravenous access secure and adequate? | | |
| Is the patient appropriately resuscitated and perfused? | | |
| Is the urine output adequate? | | |
| Is the patient haemodynamically stable? | | |
| What is the current GCS or sedation level? | | |
| What is the current pupillary response? | | |
| Are there any focal neurological signs? | | |
| Is the patient fitting? | | |
| What is the patient's core temperature prior to transfer? | | |
| Is the patient stable physiologically? | | |
| Is the patient appropriately monitored and treated? | | |
| Is the patient secure on the transfer trolley? | | |
| Does all of the portable monitoring, the transport ventilator and other equipment work after switch-over? | | |
| Any other injuries may affect safety of transfer or may adversely affected by transfer? Have they been appropriately treated? | | |
| Anything else anticipated as potential problem? | | |

Fig. 5.3   Checklist for patient preparation.

## MRI – A SPECIAL CASE

MRI is becoming commonplace in UK hospitals, and seriously ill and injured patients are often transferred from the A&E department or ITU for urgent imaging. With the advent of

| Am I ready for transfer? | Yes | Comments |
|---|---|---|
| Appropriate and warm clothing? | | |
| Spare cash? | | |
| Mobile telephone? | | |
| Telephone numbers of departure and destination hospitals? | | |
| Fed, watered and toileted? | | |
| Notify hospital switchboard and interested parties of departure? | | |
| Am I happy with myself, my team, my transport and my patient? | | |

Fig. 5.4    Personal checklist.

interventional techniques and the use of magnets of increasing strength, doctors and other health workers have the potential for increased exposure to specific MRI hazards and concerns have also been expressed over patient safety.

## Occupational hazards

The occupational hazards to which health professionals may be exposed include:

- magnetic fields,
- acoustic noise,
- unscavenged anaesthetic gases (if being used to provide general anaesthesia).

### Magnetic fields

Two types of MRI scanner are currently used in the UK:

- *Superconducting magnet* – an electric current is passed through a supercooled solenoid of wire which generates the magnetic field.

- *Permanent magnet* – the magnetic field is generated between two large fixed masses of ferromagnetic material.

The magnetic fields produced in both types of magnet consist of the following:

- *Static fields* – extend beyond the confines of the magnet but the strength depends on the configuration and shielding of the magnet. It decreases rapidly as the distance from the magnet increases.
- *Switched gradient fields* – present only within the confines of the magnet and present no hazard.
- *Radiofrequency fields* – present only within the confines of the magnet and present no hazard.

The intense static magnetic field can be demonstrated by the attraction of ferromagnetic metals towards the bore of the scanner. Apart from the obvious dangers of being injured by unrestrained objects or by the movement (or malfunction) of any MRI incompatible implants within the body, short-term exposure represents no known health risk. There are limitations on what types of equipment can be used (discuss with your MRI department), and remember that watches and electronic equipment such as calculators and pocket computers may be damaged, and credit cards or other cards with magnetic data will become unusable.

### Acoustic noise

Vibration of the switched gradient coils causes high levels of noise during scanning. These levels may reach a mean of 106 dB and an anaesthetist or other health professional remaining in the scanning room may be exposed to an average daily dose in excess of 92 dB. Hearing protection is essential during all but the shortest exposures to high-intensity noise.

## Clinical safety

MRI scanning poses additional hazards to the patient that are unrelated to the occupational hazards described above. Limitations on equipment which can be safely used in the scanner, and difficulty with monitoring conscious level and the adequacy of airway patency when patients are in the bore of the scanner (especially from a remote location) all have major implications on safety. A survey of experienced anaesthetists who regularly sedate or anaesthetize elective patients for MRI concluded that sedation in scanning rooms is unsafe, even in skilled hands. General anaesthesia, with a definitive secure airway and with appropriate monitoring, offers a safer, more certain and a more effective method of providing the necessary conditions for high-quality scans.

## THE DANGERS OF INTRAHOSPITAL PATIENT MOVEMENT

### Do no further harm!

Intrahospital transfer of patients involves an increased risk of physiological instability due to the effects of movement, vibration and variations in environmental temperature. Moving patients out of their somewhat familiar environment on the ward or the critical care unit may result in acute disorientation and confusion. In addition the patient's mood and affect may change, and he may become increasingly anxious, frightened or tearful and depressed.

The following adverse effects due to further insults on the respiratory and cardiovascular systems occur frequently during transfer, even when these patients appear relatively stable prior to movement:

- hypoxia,
- hyper- or hypocapnia,
- hyper- or hypotension.

These physiological derangements may occur in isolation or in combination. Depending on the underlying pathology, abnormalities of ventilation, inadequate perfusion or an increased cardiovascular stress response can lead to catastrophic deterioration.

Even though the transfer takes place within the confines of a hospital, there is very limited additional help available if a crisis arises. Hospital corridors and lifts provide limited space and little or no privacy. Once en route, the transfer team and the patient leave a purpose built and suitably equipped environment behind and very often the destination may be less than ideal for intensive patient care. CT or MRI scanner rooms or other investigation suites are sometimes inadequately designed and may lack appropriate, sufficient, and easily accessible medical equipment, in addition to poor access to the patient.

The transfer team relies almost entirely on self-sufficiency in terms of drugs, equipment, and manpower. Battery operated monitors, gas-driven ventilators and suction units, battery powered syringe drivers and infusion pumps, and the supply of oxygen via cylinders all have the potential to suddenly fail or malfunction.

Clearly, transfers must be kept to an absolute minimum, if the patient's condition is unstable. Whenever possible, resources should be moved to the patient rather than vice versa. There will, however, be scenarios where a patient requires an urgent investigation despite being in an immediately life-threatening condition. Depending on the outcome of the initial transfer (such as to the CT scanner), there may be a follow-up requirement for a secondary transfer (e.g. to the operating theatre). It is important to ensure that the patient may be transferred directly from one destination to the other without having to return to the initial point of origin in the meantime.

In view of the multiple dangers associated with intrahospital transfers, three overriding principles are recommended:

- The benefits must outweigh the risks.

- Dangers associated with transfers must be minimized by using staff experienced in transfer medicine or closely supervised by those who are.
- Adequate monitoring equipment should be in place and functioning.

### Who escorts the patient?

The ideal team to undertake the transfer consists of a minimum of three appropriately trained people. The level of seniority and experience of team members depends on the patient's condition and the destination of the transfer:

- *Doctor* – should be competent in resuscitation, airway care, ventilation and other organ system support.
- *Nurse, operating department assistant or practitioner (ODA/ODP)* – carries independent professional responsibility towards the patient and should be appropriately qualified and competent in the transfer procedure and nursing care required.
- *Porter* – should be familiar with the route, trolley or bed, and the oxygen cylinders.

   Others may include:

- ambulance technicians or paramedics,
- trainee – this person should be recognized as such – there to receive training and supervision until deemed competent and only then 'signed off' to undertake transfer duties unsupervised.

Anaesthetists are ideally placed for this role providing they undergo additional training in patient transportation. Specialized transfers, for instance of neonates, children, and critically injured adult patients, even within the hospital, may require advice from the appropriate speciality and they should be undertaken by experienced, trained senior specialist registrars or, ideally, by consultants. Occasionally both an anaesthetist and another specialist will be required to assist.

The nurse (or ODA/ODP) and doctor must be thoroughly familiar with all the equipment in use, the patient's current condition and the pre-arranged logistics of the transfer. There is no place for professional boundaries as far as technical, medical or nursing tasks are concerned. Only a seamless team effort will ensure a high-quality intrahospital transfer without avoidable critical incidents. Staff must have up to date knowledge in patient transportation and undergo frequent updates in safe transfer techniques. Careful selection of appropriately trained staff will ensure well-prepared, safe, and expeditious transfers.

All members of the transfer team are essential for the safe conduct of the transfer, but when a doctor is present, he will inevitably have overall responsibility for the patient (see Duty of care in Chapter 12). The team's clinical acumen, judgement, experience, and the appropriate interpretation of any information provided by monitoring equipment, together with increased situational awareness, will minimize the potential for crisis or disaster.

## Equipment and documentation

The equipment for intrahospital transfer has the same requirements as equipment for interhospital transfers. It should be

- robust,
- lightweight,
- failsafe,
- battery powered,
- portable,
- fully compatible and modular,

- illuminated displays,
- visible and audible alarms,
- user friendly.

The standard of monitoring the patient during the transfer is essentially the same as that prior to transfer. Modalities monitored depend on the condition of the patient and the likelihood of any deterioration; similarly any equipment and any drugs and infusions depend on the level of therapy the patient is currently receiving. Provision in equipment and drugs should always be made for a sudden deterioration of the patient or, in the worst case scenario, for resuscitation. Documentation of vital signs, fluid balance and any other relevant observations must be undertaken in the same way as in the ward or ICU.

Minimum standard monitoring modalities for a critically ill patient comprise:

- respiratory rate,
- oxygen saturation (pulse oximetry),
- end-tidal capnography (if intubated),
- HR,
- single lead ECG,
- non-invasive BP,
- CVP.

Other desirable modalities include:

- inspired oxygen concentration,
- invasive BP,
- urine output,
- temperature.

Yet others may be clinically indicated:

- intracranial pressure (ICP),

- blood gas analysis,
- Glasgow Coma Score (GCS).

To summarize, all monitoring that has been undertaken on the ward should be continued throughout the transfer.

In addition to a compact multi-modality monitor, preferably with an integrated defibrillator, the following major items of equipment are also essential:

- bag-valve mask device with oxygen reservoir,
- sufficient oxygen in lightweight cylinders,
- portable suction unit,
- warming blanket.

Drugs, IV fluids, resuscitation equipment including laryngo-scopes, gum-elastic bougie and a selection of endotracheal tubes are best kept in a transfer backpack. In addition, specialized equipment is required for paediatric transfers.

Depending on the destination of the intrahospital transfer, the receiving end may have monitoring equipment, a ventilator and gas supplies available. Provided these are frequently and regularly checked, a switch-over after arrival is advisable to save on batteries and cylinder oxygen supply. Battery life on items not available at the destination can be prolonged if electric cables accompany the patient, so that equipment can be connected to the mains electricity supply for as long as possible.

A dedicated transfer documentation form with threefold carbon copy (one each for the clinical notes, the nursing notes and the doctor) should be used throughout an intrahospital transfer comprising of the following sections to be completed:

- Patient details.
- Transfer details: where to and when.
- Vital signs and arterial blood gases pre-transfer.

- Any comments regarding stabilization pre-transfer.
- Staff arranging transfer and indication.
- Escorting personnel details including seniority.
- Monitoring and equipment used during transfer.
- Vital signs, observations, fluid balance, and clinical interventions during transfer.
- Special precautions taken including spinal immobilization.
- Transfer comments and problems encountered.
- Critical incidents.
- Equipment malfunction.
- Timings.
- Signature by transfer team.

Ideally intrahospital transfer documentation data should be entered into a dedicated database to enable audit of transfers undertaken, provide trainees with evidence of transfers undertaken and facilitate quality assurance.

## FURTHER READING

Intensive Care Society (1997) Guidelines for the Transport of the Critically Ill Adult. Intensive Care Society: London.

Runcie CJ (1997) Resuscitation, stabilization and preparation for transport. In: Morton NS et al. (eds) Stabilization and Transport of the Critically Ill. Churchill Livingstone: London.

Wallace PGM, Ridley SA (1999) Transport of critically ill patients. In: Singer M, Grant I (eds) ABC of Intensive Care. BMJ: London.

# 6

# Inter-ITU transfers

The frequency of interhospital transfer of patients is increasing, mostly due to the increasing complexity of health care with concentration of skills into specialized centres and the relative lack of intensive care bed availability. This chapter focuses on the transport of high dependency and intensive care patients and, although the principles of safe transport between ICUs are no different to those discussed in Chapters 4 and 5, critical care patients offer the most difficult challenges and require immense planning, preparation, skill, knowledge and teamwork to achieve success.

The aim of transfer is to improve the quality of care provided to the patient. The safe surroundings in the ambulance must attempt to mirror the attention provided in an ICU, but the transfer should at least do no harm. Even this aim is not always possible:

- over 10,000 intensive care patients are transferred annually in the UK,
- most hospitals transfer fewer than 20, too few to allow medical and nursing personnel to gain expertise,

- 90% of patients are accompanied by staff from the referring hospital,
- recommendations from the Intensive Care Society and the Association of Anaesthetists state that retrieval teams from the accepting hospital should conduct the transfer.

## HAZARDS OF TRANSPORTATION

Patient transportation is certainly a 'Cinderella' service, with most patients being escorted by on-call anaesthetic trainees. These doctors often have little experience and their departure from the referring hospital leaves it inadequately staffed.

Critically ill patients have deranged physiology and require organ support and invasive monitoring. They tolerate movement, changes in temperature and vibration poorly, and complications are not uncommon. Audits suggest that 15% of patients arrive at the destination hospital with detrimental hypoxia or hypotension, and 10% have injuries that were undetected before transfer. Complications en route may be less frequent if more senior anaesthetists accompany the patients, or if fewer personnel in specialist teams are allowed to gather experience. Once in the vehicle, supervision and advice is difficult to obtain.

## ORGANIZATION

A regional approach may allow retrieval teams to be established but, at the very least, each hospital should have

- designated consultant responsible for transfers,
- guidelines for referral and for the transfer itself,
- equipment specifically prepared and packed,
- personnel nominated to check, replenish, clean, and recharge equipment,

- nominated medical and nursing transfer personnel,
- good communication within and between hospitals,
- proper routines for referral between hospitals,
- regular audit.

### Initial communication

Poor initial communication is a frequent occurrence to which there is no easy solution. The details of the patient to be transferred must be discussed between the referring and receiving medical teams at senior (preferably consultant) level. The decision to transfer may yet to be made and advice on the feasibility of transfer may be sought. The escorting medical team must raise any valid concerns at the outset. Do not assume that any decisions already taken to transfer are the *correct* ones. Clear answers are needed for the following:

- Why is transfer occurring now?
- Is the medical risk acceptable?

Aim to gather as much information as possible. This must include history, previous treatment and operations, current care and treatment requirements, and future management plan. Modern information and communication technology enables real-time discussion and data transfer by telephone, telemetry, or via the internet, so distance (even international) is no longer a problem.

## TRANSFER DECISIONS

The timing of transfer for certain groups of patients is critical. Guidelines have been published to help the decision-making process, e.g. in head injury patients, but for others it is more difficult. For instance, in patients with multiple organ failure, the balance of risk and benefit needs to be carefully considered before the decision on whether and how to send or retrieve the patient is made.

The choice of transport mode depends on

- urgency,
- mobilization time,
- distance,
- weather,
- traffic conditions,
- cost.

Road transfer will be satisfactory for most patients but the advantages and disadvantages of different modes of transport are highlighted in Table 6.1. Vehicles must have

- trolley access and fixing systems,
- sufficient space for two or three medical attendants,
- lighting and temperature control within the cabin,
- adequate gases and electricity supply,
- storage space for drugs and equipment,
- good communications,
- sirens and warning lights.

## EQUIPMENT

General equipment issues are discussed in detail in Chapter 10, but some extra notes are important when considering intensive care patients.

### Electrical equipment

Know the machine's expected battery life and ensure they are fully charged. Most monitors have a 3–6 h published life. This is notoriously inaccurate. A shortened life occurs with age of

Table 6.1 The advantages and disadvantages of different modes of transport

| Mode | Advantages | Disadvantages |
|---|---|---|
| Road ambulance | Low cost<br>Rapid mobilization<br>Less weather<br>  dependency<br>Easier patient<br>  monitoring | Slow over long distances<br>Dependent on traffic<br>conditions |
| Helicopter air ambulance | Recommended for<br>  journeys over 50 miles<br>Fast and (possibly)<br>  direct | Slow to mobilize<br>Requires ground ambulances<br>  at either end if no dedicated<br>  hospital landing sites<br>Noisy<br>Vibration<br>Small cabin<br>Often only available during<br>  daylight<br>Expensive |
| Fixed wing air ambulance | Recommended for<br>  journeys over 150 miles<br>Compared to a<br>  helicopter:<br>  faster<br>  more space<br>  less noise and<br>    vibration<br>  less weather<br>    dependent<br>  less costly<br>  24 h service | Slow to mobilize<br>Requires ground ambulances<br>  at either end<br>Distance to nearest airport<br>  may be great |

the battery and increased electrical demands (e.g. frequent non-invasive BP cuff cycling or constant use of backlight). Spare batteries are essential.

## Multi-function units

Compact multi-function monitors are available from several leading manufacturers (e.g. Hewlett-Packard, Datex, and

Protocol). They are convenient and greatly improve patient safety but expensive (up to £12,000 per unit). An acceptable device should be capable of monitoring continuous ECG, pulse oximetry, two pressure waveforms, non-invasive BP, capnography and temperature. The ability to produce a strip-chart printout is also useful. It should have a clear display readable in a variety of lighting conditions. An orange/black display gives good clarity. Grey liquid crystal displays are difficult to read in bright light.

### Ventilators

Gas-powered fluid-logic ventilators are ideal (e.g. Dräger Oxylog series, Pneupac, and Ventipac). They are small, lightweight, reliable and robust, and need no electrical supply. Inspiratory and expiratory times are set, together with a flow rate. There is usually a choice between ventilation on 100% oxygen, or 'air-mix' (approximately 40%). The more sophisticated models have a synchronized intermittent mandatory ventilation (SIMV) mode, airway pressure alarms and a positive end expiratory pressure (PEEP) valve. Humidification must be provided via a heat/moisture exchange filter. These ventilators are suitable for children and adults with a variety of lung pathology and are able to generate a peak inspiratory pressure of 60–80 cmH$_2$0.

### Oxygen

Ventilator oxygen consumption depends on inspired oxygen fraction and MV. A 10 l min$^{-1}$ estimate is a useful starting point. A size E (640 l) oxygen cylinder will last approximately 1 h, the larger size F (1360 l) approximately 2¼ h. Oxygen failure or supply exhaustion when transporting patients with increased oxygen demand is catastrophic. Carriage of approximately twice the total calculated oxygen requirement is recommended.

## Defibrillator

Manual defibrillators (e.g. Lifepack, Laerdal, and Hewlett Packard portable models) are preferable to semi-automatic models since the electronic algorithm may in theory be confused by vibration artefact. External pacing facility is desirable.

## Syringe drivers

Syringe pumps are essential for accurate drug delivery. The double-syringe types are more compact and convenient than those taking a single syringe, but it is important to ensure that pumps and syringes are compatible.

## Doctor's bag

A comprehensive doctor's bag should contain all routine anaesthetic and emergency drugs in sufficient quantity for the entire transfer. Several manufacturers make custom-designed emergency bags for the ambulance and mountain rescue services. These are ideal. There should be ample storage space for drugs, together with a variety of compartments for essential airway equipment, cannulae, syringes, IV fluid, chest drain sets (with underwater seal kit or Heimlich valve), and sundry items such as gloves, swabs, tape, sharps box, and so on. An inventory of drugs and equipment is essential for checking contents and recording expiry dates.

## THE MEDICAL TEAM

Successful interhospital transfer requires a well-coordinated team effort. A full-time hospital consultant in anaesthesia or intensive care medicine should be responsible for the service, training of transfer personnel and audit of transfer activities. In addition to the crew of the ambulance, a critically ill patient should be accompanied by a minimum of two attendants:

- Doctor, usually an anaesthetist trained in intensive care with
  - previous transfer experience,
  - at least 2 years postgraduate experience,
  - at least a primary qualification in the specialty.
- Assisted by a qualified anaesthetic or intensive care nurse, paramedic, or technician familiar with intensive care procedures and equipment.

## FINAL PREPARATION

Stabilization of the patient should follow the principles outlined by the ABC approach in Chapter 3 and, since hypovolaemic patients tolerate movement poorly, circulating volume should be normal or supranormal before departure. IV loading will usually be required to maintain satisfactory blood pressure, perfusion and urine output, but inotrope therapy may also be needed. Particularly unstable patients may need CVP or pulmonary artery pressure monitoring to optimize filling pressures and cardiac output. In addition, monitoring immediately prior to transfer should include ECG and blood gas analysis.

Documentation must include a referral letter, the clinical notes, X-rays, and results of all investigations. Any cross-matched blood or blood products must accompany the patient. Finally, the receiving ITU consultant and nurse-in-charge must be informed of the estimated time of arrival and travel arrangements should be discussed with relatives.

## THE TRANSFER

If possible, the patient should be positioned to provide maximum access during the transfer. Allow space at the head-end to allow monitoring and management of the airway. All round access is ideal but seldom achievable in UK ambulances, and all but impossible in aircraft.

The transfer should be undertaken smoothly and rarely at high speed. The staff/patient ratio during the journey is better than normally expected in the hospital ITU and the aim is to provide the same standard of monitoring, nursing care and medical intervention. The caveat, of course, is that in transit it can be almost impossible to undertake major procedures. Any significant incidents may be best managed after the ambulance has pulled over to the side of the road (a luxury not available in aircraft).

## SPECIALIZED CRITICAL CARE TRANSFERS

Specialized coronary care transport teams have been operating in the USA since the 1980s and, although it is recognized that America has widely differing patient transport needs because of vast distances between hospitals, it is likely that similar schemes will operate out of the UK in the future. Recent advances in intra-aortic balloon counterpulsation (IABC) technology have made transport of selected patients safer. Accepted indications for transfer of a patient on an IABC pump are given in Table 6.2.

Table 6.2    Indications for IABC transport

Accelerating angina (patient transport to a cardiac facility for bypass surgery)
Ischaemic or idiopathic cardiomyopathy when cardiac transplantation is an
  option
Emergency surgical repair of structural defects, such as mitral valve defect
Haemodynamic instability during a cardiac catheterization
Need for advanced pharmacological therapy necessitating transfer to a tertiary
  care facility
IABC pump-dependent patient has exhausted the resources of the referring
  facility

Source: Mertlich G, Quaal SJ (1989) Air transport of the patient requiring intra-aortic balloon pumping. Crit Care Nurs Clin North Am 1(3): 443.

Haemofiltration in transit is a controversial issue. Even though the RAF pioneered the international aeromedical transfer of renal dialysis patients in the 1960s, civilian practice has not followed. However, new haemofiltration technology may eventually prove small and robust enough to be useful for long international flights.

## FURTHER READING

A group of neurosurgeons (1984) Guidelines for the initial management after head injury in adults. BMJ 288: 983–985.

Association of Anaesthetists of Great Britain and Ireland (2000) Recommendations for standards of monitoring during anaesthesia and recovery. AAGBI: London.

Donelly JA, McGinn GH (1997) Equipment for the transfer of the critically ill. In: Morton NS et al. (eds) Stabilization and Transport of the Critically Ill. Churchill Livingstone: London.

Intensive Care Society (1997) Guidelines for the Transport of the Critically Ill Adult. Intensive Care Society: London.

Mertlich G, Quaal SJ (1989) Air transport of the patient requiring intra-aortic balloon pumping. Crit Care Nurs Clin North Am 1(3): 443.

Neuroanaesthesia Society of Great Britain and Ireland (1996) Recommendations for the Transfer of Patients with Acute Head Injuries to Neurosurgical Units. AAGBI: London.

Wallace PGM, Ridley SA (1999) Transport of critically ill patients. In: Singer M, Grant I (eds) ABC of Intensive Care. BMJ: London.

# 7

# Clinical considerations in specialized transport

## TRANSPORT OF PATIENTS WITH HEAD INJURY OR INTRACRANIAL HAEMORRHAGE

Ten thousand of the one million patients who attend hospital in the UK with head trauma each year have an injury that merits transfer to a regional neurosurgical unit. These regional centres may be many miles from the admitting hospital and modern neurosurgical services are geared towards identifying patients at risk of intracranial haematoma and transferring them urgently for definitive care. Neurosurgical literature is full of warnings about delays in treatment of intracranial bleeds, but there are dangers of transportation if the transfer is undertaken by an ill-prepared team or with an unstable patient. The need to resuscitate and stabilize patients prior to departure is as important, if not more so, than the rapid transfer itself. Criteria for neurosurgical referral (Table 7.1) are well established in the UK, but the receiving consultant needs certain information before advising on the need and timing of the transfer (Table 7.2).

**Table 7.1    UK criteria for neurosurgical referral**

*Immediately after initial assessment and resuscitation*
  Fractured skull with
    any alteration in level of consciousness (GCS <15)
    or focal neurological signs
    or fits
    or any other neurological symptoms
  No skull fracture seen
    coma persisting after resuscitation
    deterioration in level of consciousness (GCS <15)
    focal pupil or limb signs
*Urgent, but not necessarily immediate*
  Compound depressed fracture
  Penetrating head injury
  CSF leak from nose or ear
  Confusion persisting for more than 6 h
  Persistent or worsening headache or vomiting

**Table 7.2    Information required by receiving consultant before advising on the need and timing of the transfer**

| | |
|---|---|
| Patient's age and past medical history | Injuries |
| History of injury | Skull fracture |
| Time | Extracranial injuries |
| Cause/mechanism | Management so far |
| Neurological state | Airway protection and ventilation |
| Level of consciousness on | Circulatory status and IV therapy |
| arrival | First aid treatment and associated |
| Talked or not since injury | injuries |
| Trend in level of consciousness | Monitoring |
| Pupil and limb responses | Drug and times of administration |
| Cardiorespiratory state | |
| BP and HR | |
| Arterial blood gases | |
| Respiratory rate and pattern | |

## Patient preparation

The major consideration for any patient suffering neurological injury is to prevent secondary damage by cerebral hypoxia and

Table 7.3   The GCS

| Eye opening response | | Best verbal response | | Best motor response (upper limb) | |
|---|---|---|---|---|---|
| 4 | Spontaneous | 5 | Orientated | 6 | Obeys commands |
| 3 | To speech | 4 | Confused | 5 | Localizes to pain |
| 2 | To pain | 3 | Inappropriate words | 4 | Normal flexion to pain |
| 1 | None | 2 | Incomprehensible sounds | 3 | Spastic flexion to pain |
| | | 1 | None | 2 | Extension to pain |
| | | | | 1 | None |

the effects of cerebral compression. The GCS (Table 7.3) should therefore be documented in the notes before departure. A decrease of more than two points is highly suggestive of serious neurological deterioration and constitutes a neurosurgical emergency.

An IV cannula should be inserted for the prophylactic or therapeutic management of nausea, vomiting, and seizures. The conscious head-injured patient is more prone to nausea and motion sickness, and an anti-emetic may be recommended to prevent the elevated ICP that accompanies vomiting and retching. Most anti-emetics affect alertness, potentially making the GCS unreliable. On advice from the receiving neurosurgical consultant, mannitol may be administered to decrease ICP by initiating a diuresis, and thiopentone may be used to further lower resistant elevated ICP and cerebral oxygen demand.

Known epileptics require premedication prior to departure, either by an increase in their normal anticonvulsant therapy, or with a benzodiazepine. Patients known to be at risk of having seizures should travel on a stretcher and convulsions that occur must be stopped to prevent further cerebral damage. Convulsing patients must

- have a secure and patent airway,
- receive 100% oxygen,

- be kept warm,
- be protected from self-harm.

## Cerebral monitoring

Complex techniques such as transcranial doppler sonography, near infrared spectroscopy and jugular venous oxygen saturation are available in many neuro intensive care units, but the equipment is too bulky and not robust enough to use in an ambulance. Standard ITU monitoring (Chapter 6) is essential to prevent secondary brain injury, but ICP monitoring is often available, especially if there is a delay in initiating the transfer, or if a multiply injured patient is admitted in the first instance to a general ITU for stabilization. Modern ICP probes are easily inserted through a small drill hole and give reliable recordings wherever the transducer is sited. They use a liquid crystal display compatible with routine multi-modal monitor displays, but monitoring ICP alone is not as useful as cerebral perfusion pressure (CPP), where CPP equals mean arterial BP minus ICP.

## The dangers of aeromedical transport

Air in the cranium will expand at altitude and any patient who has had a craniotomy should not fly before the 7th postoperative day unless the aircraft is pressurized to the altitude of the site where the operation was performed. Similar care is necessary after an air encephalogram or ventriculogram, penetrating head injury, or in the presence of cerebrospinal fluid (CSF) leakage from the ears or nose. If a CSF leak is present at ground level, it will drain slightly faster at altitude.

## Associated injuries

### Spinal injury

Cervical spine injury is associated with significant head trauma and fractures of the clavicle and the first or second ribs. In the presence of such a history, suitable protection of the cervical spine is essential even if a fracture or subluxation has not been diagnosed. Up to 15% of cervical fractures are missed on initial X-rays.

## Facial injuries

All patients with severe facial injuries should be considered to have a base of skull fracture until proven otherwise and the team must be alert for compromise of airway patency. Any patient who has external fixation of the jaws must have either a quick-release device fitted to the apparatus or have wire or band cutters easily accessible. Prior to the start of the transfer, patients with facial and mandibular immobilization should be given an anti-emetic by intramuscular or IV injection, and a NG or orogastric tube should be sited. Patients with unstable midface fractures awaiting definitive correction are likely to require intubation with an uncut endotracheal tube (because of facial swelling) and packing of the posterior pharynx to prevent secondary haemorrhage.

## Subarachnoid haemorrhage

Rebleeding from an acute subarachnoid haemorrhage is common. Recommended times for patient transfer after the acute event are either during the first 48 h or after 2 weeks have elapsed.

## TRANSPORT OF PATIENTS WITH SPINAL INJURIES

### Pathophysiological problems

Normal physiology may be grossly deranged after spinal cord injury – the exact nature depends on the level and severity of the damage.

- Paralysis of intercostal muscles and the diaphragm impairs ventilation and leads to hypoxia. Any accompanying chest injuries exacerbate the situation. A pulmonary assessment is essential to ensure that those patients requiring supplemental oxygen or ventilation are identified, appropriately managed and closely monitored.

- High thoracic and cervical spine injury to the sympathetic chain results in the combination of unopposed vagal (parasympathetic) stimulation and loss of vascular tone. This is neurogenic shock, pathognomically characterized by hypotension in the presence of bradycardia. Venous pooling exacerbates the pathophysiologic effect of any true fluid losses. IV access is essential before the journey is started.

- The lack of vagal opposition produces a bradycardia which may progress to asystole when the vagus is further stimulated by the placement of an oropharyngeal or nasopharyngeal airway, NG tube, or urinary catheter. Atropine is a potent parasympatholytic agent which can be administered prior to these procedures, and the ECG should be monitored throughout the transfer.

- The spinal patient is at increased risk of PE, the incidence being greatest during the 2nd and 3rd weeks after injury. Unless contraindicated, patients should be stabilized on anticoagulant therapy prior to departure. Those not already anticoagulated should receive 5,000 units of heparin subcutaneously before transfer. Elastic stockings decrease the risk of deep venous thrombosis.

- Vasomotor lability and sensory deficits prevent adequate thermoregulation, and patients may be liable to both hypothermia and heat intolerance. Ensure that the internal temperature of the ambulance or aircraft is comfortable for the patient, and protect him from excess heat or cold when out of the vehicle.

- Paralysis and impaired sensation predispose to pressure sores, especially in the presence of hypoperfused and hypoxic tissues. Ensure that the patient is lying on a soft, smooth surface, and remove any hard objects or intrusions.

Soft fluid packs over the heels and ankles or sheep-skin booties are helpful, but no substitute for frequent movement of the patient to disperse the load onto other areas.

## Prehospital transport of spinal patients

In the primary transfer of spinal patients to hospital, those at risk of cervical injury should have the neck and back immobilized on a rigid spine board and supported in the neutral position. This is best done with a hard collar and 'head huggers', foam blocks or rolled towels placed on either side of the head. Tape should be placed over the forehead to secure the head to a spinal board or the stretcher upon which the patient is lying (Figure 7.1). A vacuum mattress-type neck collar may also be used, but all air must be evacuated from the collar.

A scoop (clamshell) stretcher is useful for safely transferring patients between stretcher types and between stretchers and

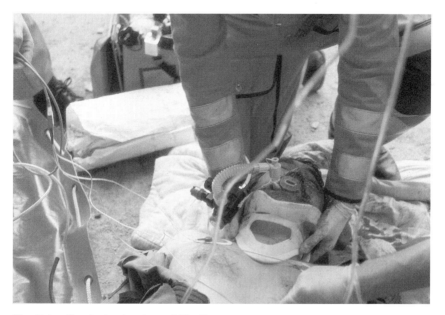

Fig. 7.1 Cervical spine immobilization.

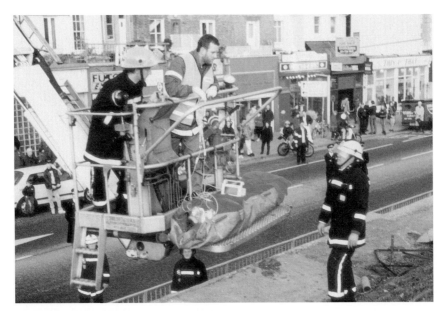

Fig. 7.2    Transport on a vacuum mattress.

beds, but extrication devices (such as the Kendrick and Russell devices), although useful during the release of entrapped patients at complex trauma scenarios, are unsuitable for the transfer of patients.

### Secondary transfer of spinal patients

- If the journey is likely to be long, the patient will need to be safely turned. Simple arrangements include periodically turning the board/patient unit from side to side, but transport on a vacuum mattress, conformed to the patient's body contours and lined with a sheepskin blanket (Figure 7.2), is safer and more comfortable.
- Stryker and Povey frames (Figure 7.3) are too heavy and bulky for most ambulances, and need a lifting device for emplanement on large aircraft. The prone position should not be used because of diaphragmatic splinting which reduces ventilation.

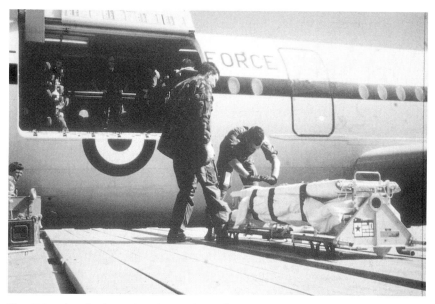

Fig. 7.3 A spinal turning frame (Povey) occasionally used for long–duration transfers.

- Patients whose cervical spine has already been stabilized may well have traction tongs in situ. Crutchfield's and Cone's tongs are the most suitable for transport. Closed systems are essential; free hanging weights are dangerous and unreliable.
- Stomach gas may splint the diaphragm and impede adequate ventilation, and cause regurgitation with possible aspiration. A freely draining NG tube should be placed before departure.
- Urinary catheterization, even if only for the duration of the transfer, prevents the problems of urinary incontinence for both patient and medical team. A further advantage is the ability to measure hourly urine output as a guide to the adequacy of circulating volume.
- Conscious patients with spinal injuries require enormous reassurance, tact, and psychological support. Resist the temptation to enter into discussion about the likely outcome of the patient's injuries.

## TRANSPORT OF BURNED PATIENTS

Burns of less than 15% body surface area (BSA) will generally not cause haemodynamic instability during transfer, but patients with small burns may still require movement to a specialist unit. The American Burns Association referral guidelines are given in Table 7.4, and a scheme for assessing BSA burned is illustrated in Figure 7.4. These transfers require careful thought and planning. For instance, patients with airway burns will require intubation and ventilation, burned hands may mean that a patient cannot look after himself, whereas burned feet or perineum may mean the patient cannot walk. Even for clinically insignificant burns, patients being transported on commercial airlines may not be allowed to travel if their appearance is considered to be potentially distressing to other passengers. Large surface area burns pose special problems in transportation but methodical stabilization with careful packaging will do much to prevent problems occurring en route. The issues of concern are best considered using an ABC approach.

**Table 7.4   The American Burns Association criteria for transfer to a specialist Burns Unit**

Full thickness burn >5% BSA in any age group
Partial thickness and full thickness burns
  >10% BSA in age under 10s and over 50s
  >20% BSA in other age groups
Inhalation injury
Burns of
  face (especially eyes and ears)
  hands and feet
  genitalia and perineum
  overlying major joints
Electrical burns and lightning injury
Significant chemical burns
In the presence of
  pre-existing illness or concurrent trauma that might affect
    mortality or morbidity
  special social emotional or rehabiltative problems

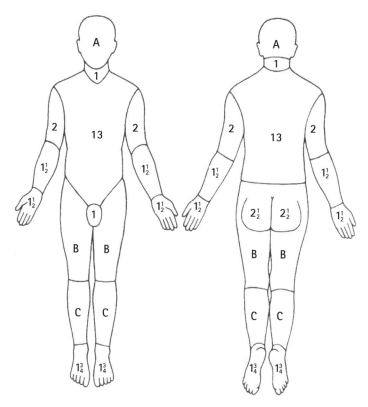

Plot the areas of full and partial thickness burn: ignore areas of simple erythema and superficial sooting

### Approximate changes in BSA with age

| Area | Represents | Age (years) | | | | | |
|---|---|---|---|---|---|---|---|
| | | <1 | 1–4 | 5–9 | 10–14 | Adolescent | Adult |
| A | ½ of head | 9½ | 8½ | 6½ | 5½ | 4½ | 3½ |
| B | ½ of 1 thigh | 2¾ | 3¼ | 4 | 4½ | 4½ | 4¾ |
| C | ½ of 1 lower leg | 2½ | 2½ | 2¾ | 3 | 3¼ | 3½ |

Fig. 7.4   The Lund–Browder chart – a scheme for assessing % BSA burned.

## Airway

Oedema of the airway and neck can occur rapidly, causing direct and indirect airway obstruction and distortion of normal landmarks. Elective intubation with an uncut oral endotracheal tube is essential in patients with suspected respiratory tract burn. If intubation is not possible, a surgical airway will be required but the distortion of normal anatomy can be problematic. The following features are suggestive of respiratory burn:

- facial burns,
- carbonaceous sputum,
- singeing of nasal hairs and eyebrows,
- decreased conscious level.

## Breathing

In addition to direct respiratory damage, significant burn injuries increase the basal metabolic rate and therefore also oxygen demand. Patients with problems of oxygenation or pulmonary function must be identified well before departure so that adequate oxygen supplements, mechanical ventilation, or other special requirements can be met. Tracheostomy tubes, unless newly inserted, should be replaced prior to a long journey to minimize the risk of obstruction by mucous plugging. A spare tube should be carried.

### During transfer
- Oxygen saturation must be monitored continuously, remembering it may be inaccurate in the presence of carbon monoxide poisoning.
- End-tidal $CO_2$ measurement will help ensure adequacy of ventilation.
- Frequent, careful, aseptic suction of the airway may be required.
- Use humidified oxygen.
- Nebulized bronchodilators should be available for those with bronchospasm.
- The patient should be nursed head up.

Table 7.5  The ATLS recommended fluid regime for burns

| | |
|---|---|
| Fluid recommended | Ringer lactate (Hartmann's solution) |
| Formula | 2–4 mL/kg body weight per 1% BSA burned in 24 h |
| Regime | half in first 8 h after injury, half in the next 16 h |
| Monitoring | aim for urine output of 30–50 mL/h in adults and 1.0 mL/kg/h in children under 30 kg |

## Circulation

Considerable fluid may be lost through the burn and yet more fluid may leak into the surrounding tissues. In addition to normal maintenance, patients will need additional fluids to replace these losses and to prevent shock. A suitable fluid regime, such as the advanced trauma life support (ATLS) recommended formula (Table 7.5) should be commenced before departure. The following should be ensured:

- Secure venous access (at least two wide bore cannulae).
- Central line for further access and CVP measurement.
- A urinary catheter for hourly urine output measurement.

*During transfer*
- Whenever possible the ECG and BP should be monitored continuously.
- The urine output should be maintained at atleast 0.5–1 mL/kg/h by adjusting replacement fluid.
- Forced diuresis may be necessary for oliguria due to haemoglobinuria or myoglobinuria.
- During a transfer in an aircraft pressurized cabin, extra fluids may be required to compensate for additional evaporation in the low humidity cabin air.

## General considerations

*Pre-transfer investigations*
Before departure, patients with extensive burns or respiratory involvement should have the following investigations, and

significant abnormalities should be corrected before departure:

- arterial blood gases,
- carboxyhaemoglobin,
- haemoglobin (Hb, should be greater than 7.5 g/dL if air transportation is being considered),
- electrolytes (hyperkalaemia may occur in the presence of extensive tissue necrosis and will be worsened, perhaps catastrophically, if suxamethonium is used for rapid sequence induction).

### Escharotomy

Escharotomies should be considered if the patient has fresh deep circumferential chest or limb burns which may compromise respiration or circulation. Deep burns are painless and anaesthesia is not necessary, but decisions must be made early because bleeding will be excessive once vascular engorgement occurs. The incision is made down to fat in the centre of the burn and extended along the line of the limb or trunk (Figure 7.5). Pain indicates an area of superficial burn where no further escharotomy is necessary. Avoid exposure of tendons, vessels or nerves, and bleeding should be controlled before departure.

### Dressings

If the journey time is expected to be long, wounds should be redressed under sterile conditions prior to transfer – the inside of an ambulance or aircraft cannot guarantee sterility. En route, additional dressings can be placed over the original sterile dressing without need to further disturb the wound.

### Analgesia and sedation
- Normal ITU procedures apply to intubated patients.
- Pain relief in conscious patients is best achieved by titration with IV opiates.
- IV chlorpromazine is a useful sedative which also potentiates analgesia and has anti-emetic effects.

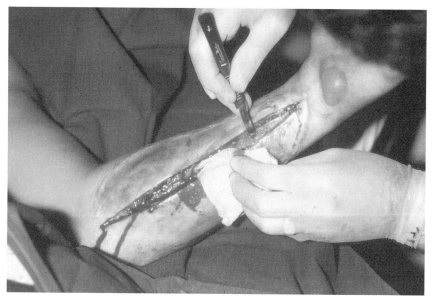

Fig. 7.5   Escharotomy – the incision is extended along the line of the limb or trunk.

*Reducing catabolism*
The metabolic rate is increased in severe burns and catabolism can be reduced by normalization of the patient's environment. This includes:

- *Temperature* – fluid loss through the burn will lead to additional heat loss through evaporation. The burn should be kept covered to prevent excess evaporation at all times. A 'space' blanket may be helpful.
- *Nutrition* – on a very long journey, anabolism must be promoted by adequate provision of calories. Dietary requirements should be calculated before transfer and given intravenously or orally as appropriate via a proven and trusted line or NG tube.

## TRANSPORT OF OBSTETRIC PATIENTS

The goal is to optimize medical care during the transport of two patients rather than one. Transport may be essential for a mother who is at risk from a medical emergency, but clearly the best and safest intensive care environment for a sick or very pre-term foetus is the uterus. With the advent of high-definition ultrasound scanning in pregnancy, many congenital abnormalities are now diagnosed in the antenatal period, and the decision on where the baby should be delivered may be made in the light of the expected need for specialist neonatal, paediatric or surgical care. This has increased the need for transportation during pregnancy.

### Differences in maternal anatomy and physiology

Amongst the many changes in anatomy and physiology that occur with pregnancy, mechanical effects of the enlarging uterus cause most problems:

- Partial obstruction of the inferior vena cava and descending aorta when the woman lies flat results in supine hypotension. This is usually resolved by placing the patient on her left side, or inserting a wedge or pillow under the right hip during transfer.
- Vascular congestion of the lower limbs increases the risk of venous thrombosis and thrombophlebitis.
- Diaphragmatic compression causes a reduction in tidal volume.
- Compression of the bladder leads to frequency of micturition.

Other significant changes in pregnancy include:

- *Haematological* – an increase in plasma volume, a slight increase in red cell mass and a relatively raised white cell count. The pregnant woman may lose up to 1500 mL blood without signs of shock, although the foetus may already be adversely affected.

- *Hypercoaguability* – due to an overall increase in clotting factors, fibrinogen, and plasminogen inhibitor.
- *Prolonged gastric emptying* – with increased risk of regurgitation and aspiration.

### Foetal monitoring

Foetal well-being can be monitored indirectly either using a cardiotocogram or by listening to foetal heart sounds. Cardiotocography is difficult and impractical during transfer, not least because of the size of most machines, but the foetal heart may be heard using Doppler from 14–16 weeks or a stethoscope from about 20 weeks. A Doppler will generally be required in transit because of the noisy environment of the ambulance, helicopter or aircraft.

### Who should supervise the patient en route?

If a patient has a life-threatening condition such as serious bleeding or severe hypertension, the accompanying doctor must be competent in resuscitation and critical care in addition to his knowledge of obstetrics. In less serious transfers it is unusual to require the presence of an obstetrician, and the skills of a competent midwife will usually suffice. However, where there is a possibility of the birth of a seriously compromised baby (e.g. under 34 weeks gestation or known to have an abnormality which may require special resuscitation from birth), a neonatal paediatrician should also be in attendance. If the transfer is by air, the escorting team should be experienced and knowledgeable about the effects of altitude on mother and foetus.

### The effect of altitude on the pregnant patient

The $FIO_2$ up to a cabin pressure of 7500 ft (normal commercial aircraft) will be sufficient to satisfy the demands of the mother and a healthy baby. Supplemental oxygen should be given to the

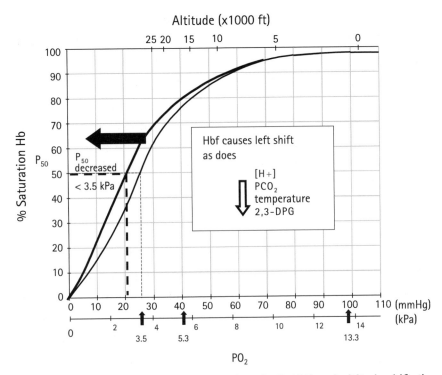

**Fig. 7.6**   Oxygen dissociation curve to show both HbF and altitude shift the curve to the left.

mother if there is any possibility that the foetus is at risk from hypoxia. Foetal haemoglobin (HbF) has a greater affinity for oxygen than its adult counterpart, and both HbF and altitude shift the oxygen dissociation curve to the left (Figure 7.6). The lower $PO_2$ in an aircraft cabin therefore facilitates oxygen delivery to the baby, but hinders its release into the baby's tissues.

## Specific problems in obstetric transfers

### In utero transfers

It is now widely recognized that the best way to transport a potentially very sick neonate is in utero so that the baby has access to neonatal intensive care immediate after birth. These types of transfer have increased with the advent of high-resolution antenatal ultrasound. Diagnoses include extreme prematurity, multiple births and any serious congenital abnormality that will require immediate treatment. Many transfers therefore involve a relatively well mother, but there is potential for a very sick baby, or worse, a baby being delivered on the journey. Close collaboration between the referring obstetric team and receiving obstetric and paediatric teams, must take place well in advance of the anticipated date of delivery to ensure such transfers take place in a timely manner.

## Vaginal bleeding

Despite the fact that many of the reasons for vaginal bleeding occur in early pregnancy, the majority that require transportation occur in the third trimester. Life-threatening causes at this time include placenta praevia, placental abruption and post-partum haemorrhage. Active fluid resuscitation and blood products may be required en route, in addition to specific therapy for the condition.

## Pre-term labour

Interhospital transfers of mothers in pre-term labour are uncommon in the UK. The proximity of mainland hospitals and the quality of facilities available at the majority make the risk of delivery during transfer unacceptable. If labour is definitely established patients should remain in the referring hospital until delivery. The neonate should then be resuscitated and stabilized before transfer, preferably accompanied by the mother. If a pre-term transfer is deemed necessary, familiarity with the administration of tocolytics, such as IV $\beta2$ sympathomimetic agents, nifedipine and possibly magnesium sulphate, is essential. Plans should be made for the unexpected delivery of the infant, particularly in terms of patient positioning, management of foetal malposition and availability of both equipment and personnel for neonatal resuscitation.

## Pre-eclampsia and eclampsia

This syndrome, characterized by hypertension and proteinuria (pre-eclampsia) and with convulsions (eclampsia) may be life threatening to both mother and baby. The treatment can be complex and may include IV magnesium sulphate, antihypertensives and anticonvulsants. Although typically occurring in pregnancy, pre-eclampsia and eclampsia may also occur for several weeks post-partum. It is crucial that the patient is accompanied by an escort capable of dealing with any eclamptic emergency that may arise. Generally, this would mean a doctor experienced in obstetric critical care.

## FURTHER READING

A group of neurosurgeons (1984) Guidelines for the initial management after head injury in adults. BMJ 288: 983–985.

American College of Surgeons Committee on Trauma (1996) ATLS Course Manual. American College of Surgeons: Chicago.

Baack BR, Smoot EC, Kucan JO et al. (1991) Helicopter transport of the patient with acute burns. J Burn Care Rehabil 12: 229–233.

Clarke JA (1982) A Colour Atlas of Burn Injuries. Chapman & Hall: London.

Elliot JP, O'Keeffe DF, Freeman RK (1982) Helicopter transportation of patients with obstetric emergencies in an urban area. Am J Obst Gynecol 143: 157–162.

Elliott JP, Sipp TL, Balazs KT (1992) Maternal transport of patients with advanced cervical dilatation – to fly or not to fly? Obst Gynecol 79: 380–382.

Gentleman D, Jennett B (1981) Hazards of inter-hospital transfer of comatose head-injured patients. Lancet 2: 853–855.

Gentleman D (1997) Head injury. In: Morton NS, Murray MP, Wallace PGM (eds) Stabilization and Transport of the Critically Ill. Churchill Livingstone: London.

Gentleman D et al. (1993) Guidelines for resuscitation and transfer of patients with serious head injury. BMJ 307: 547–552.

Grundy D, Russell J, Swain A (1990) ABC of Spinal Cord Injury. BMJ: London.

Houghton GR (1989) Spine Injuries. Gower Medical Publishing: London.

Judkins KC (1988) Aeromedical transfer of burned patients: a review with special reference to European civilian practice. Burn Incl Ther Injury 14(3): 171–179.

Low RB et al. (1988) Emergency air transport of pregnant patients: the national experience. J Emergency Med 6: 41–48.

Martin TE (2001) The oxygen dissociation curve. In: Comprehensive Trauma Nursing. Churchill Livingstone: London.

Neuroanaesthesia Society of Great Britain and Ireland (1996) Recommendations for the Transfer of Patients with Acute Head Injuries to Neurosurgical Units. AAGBI: London.

Parer JT (1982) Effects of hypoxia on the mother and fetus with emphasis on maternal air transport. Am J Obst Gyneco 142: 957–961.

Settle JAD (1986) Burns – the First Five Days. Smith & Nephew: Romford.

Staniforth P (1994) Head injuries – to be transferred or not? Injury 25: 491–492.

# 8

# Transport of paediatric patients

A child's response to illness and injury is often different to that of an adult, and appropriate management requires specialist paediatric knowledge and a new set of skills. This is well known to paediatric ICU, many of whom have their own transport (retrieval) teams.

The range of children's weights and sizes, and their physical differences, may have a bearing on transport requirements both in logistical considerations and in terms of preparation of equipment and medications.

Neonates (babies within the first month of life) are commonly transported to and from specialist units. Whilst sharing some of the problems of older children, they have their own special pathologies and needs, even further removed from the problems of adults. Many of these babies are critically ill and it is usual for a suitably trained neonatal paediatrician and neonatal nurse to accompany them. In some areas of the world, the transportation of the newborn is almost considered a specialty in its own right.

## PREHOSPITAL VERSUS INTER- OR INTRAHOSPITAL TRANSPORTATION

The same principles and logistics apply for children as for adults (Chapter 3), but there are a number of problems in prehospital paediatric management which are not so significant in adults:

- There are fewer professionals skilled in prehospital paediatric medical management.
- Comprehensive paediatric equipment may not be readily available.
- Children can deteriorate faster than adults, e.g. respiratory obstruction may occur more rapidly because of the small diameter of the airways.

A 'scoop and run' policy may therefore be appropriate at an *earlier stage* in the sick child, although adequate oxygenation before leaving the scene is still essential. If this is not possible, immediate and rapid transportation to definitive care is mandatory.

## SECONDARY TRANSPORTATION

During secondary transfer (inter- or intrahospital), as with adults, the child's condition should be optimized before moving, although undue delay should be avoided once the decision has been made. The concept of 'an intensive care bed on the move' indicates the quality of care expected from good paediatric intensive care transportation. With interhospital transfers, the details of the patient must be discussed between the referring and receiving medical teams at consultant level. Full details of the history, current therapy, and planned management should be discussed before departure (see Chapter 6).

## Who should supervise the child en route?

The bottom line is that the person or team who accompany the child must be trained and competent to deal with any problem that could arise during the time the child is en route. For the critically ill child, generally this means a senior doctor and trained paediatric intensive care nurse.

## DIFFERENCES BETWEEN ADULTS AND CHILDREN

Children die for different reasons than adults. For example, under the age of 1 year, cot death is commonest, beyond that, trauma and other emergencies, such as drowning and poisoning, predominate. Cardiac arrest is often heralded by bradycardia and is usually a terminal event resulting from hypoxia and acidosis, most commonly from an underlying respiratory cause. Resuscitation and supportive care must therefore include meticulous attention to oxygenation. Other anatomical and physiological differences are best addressed by the familiar scheme of Airway (and cervical spine), Breathing and Circulation.

### Airway

The child's airway differs from adults:

- Large tongue, big tonsils, and wobbly teeth.
- High anterior larynx.
- The cricoid cartilage is the narrowest point of the airway.
- The angle at the carina is more symmetrical.
- The upper airways are narrow and short.
- Infants less than 6 months old are obligate nasal breathers.

The practical implications during transport are as follows:

- They may be more difficult to intubate and a special (straight bladed) laryngoscope may be required.

If an intubated child is being transported the attending doctor must be confident in his ability to manage the airway of the child and reintubate if required.

- Endotracheal tubes become displaced very easily (because of the short trachea) and constant vigilance is required to ensure that the tube does not become dislodged or impinge upon the carina when the patient is moved. Tubes should be secured extremely carefully. Elective nasal intubation before departure increases tube stability.

- The narrow airway of the child can block more easily than an adult's. If increased airway swelling is possible during the journey (for instance respiratory burns and croup), elective intubation should be undertaken before departure. Intubating a child with an obstructed airway may be extremely difficult in optimum conditions and failure to secure the airway before departure may be catastrophic.

- Endotracheal tubes also block easily with secretions because of their narrow diameter. Check that suction catheters have a bore small enough to go down whichever tube has been used. They may not be part of the 'stock' supply on every ambulance or airway management box.

## Breathing

There are significant differences in children's breathing when compared to adults:

- The respiratory rate is higher than in adults (Table 8.1).
- The chest wall is very compliant. Serious internal injury may occur without rib fractures or external signs.
- Infants rely mainly on diaphragmatic breathing. They are likely to tire easily as they have fewer Type 1 (fatigue resistant) muscle fibres than an adult.

Table 8.1   Respiratory changes with age

| Age (years) | Breaths (per min) |
| --- | --- |
| Less than 2 | 30–40 |
| 2–5 | 25–30 |
| 5–12 | 20–25 |
| Over 12 | 15–20 |

- The lower airways of children are small so, in much the same way as the upper airways, they are prone to blocking with mucus plugs and secretions.

These differences are significant when transporting a very sick or injured child:

- If a small child or baby is working hard at breathing, the extra-stress of the journey may be enough to cause exhaustion and a respiratory arrest. If there is any possibility of the situation deteriorating to the point where intubation will be required on the journey, it is essential that it is undertaken before leaving.
- With a suspicious history, serious internal chest injury must be sought, even in the absence of fractures or severe bruising. Appropriate stabilization should be achieved before leaving the referring unit. This is particularly important where air transportation is to be undertaken.

## Circulation

As with adults the aim is for stabilization before leaving the referring unit. However, a number of specific differences in children must be considered:

- The pulse rate and BP vary with age (Table 8.2).

Table 8.2    Cardiovascular changes with age

| Age (years) | HR (beats/min) | Systolic BP (mmHg) |
|---|---|---|
| <2 | 110–160 | 70–90 |
| 2–5 | 95–140 | 80–100 |
| 5–12 | 80–120 | 90–110 |
| More than 12 | 60–100 | 100–120 |

NB   Systolic = 80 + (2 × age),   Diastolic = 2/3 × syotolic.

- Children compensate well for hypovolaemia. Hypotension is often not seen until 25% of the circulating volume is lost. Pulse rate and capillary refill will be abnormal before BP falls.
- BP can be technically difficult to measure on young children in the out-of-hospital setting unless it is being measured invasively.
- Childen lose heat quickly and capillary refill may be inaccurate if the child is cold. It is preferable to assess skin perfusion on the sternum or forehead rather than the fingers or toes.
- Vascular access may be very difficult, particularly in toddlers.
- Fluid input and output must be measured accurately in children and babies. Total blood volume of a 6-month-old baby is likely to be less than 500 mL.

The following considerations need to be borne in mind when undertaking a transfer of a seriously ill child with circulatory problem:

- Secure IV access at a minimum of two sites is essential. Ensure the availability of an intraosseous needle in case of an emergency in transit. If a child is significantly haemodynamically unstable, a central venous line should be inserted before departure.

- All haemodynamically unstable, ventilated children should have invasive BP monitoring. Non-invasive methods may be very difficult to undertake accurately in transit.
- All fluids should be administered via an infusion pump or syringe. Microdroppers do not run well in transit and should be avoided. In young children and babies where low-infusion rates can be expected, 50 mL syringe pumps are particularly useful, because they take up less space than standard infusion sets.
- Strict measurement of all fluid input and output must be documented on the journey.

## Neuro (disability) and exposure

Convulsions should be controlled prior to transport in the usual way. Management of coma must include optimization of blood gases, temperature, and biochemistry. In addition the following should be borne in mind:

- Children are very prone to hypoglycaemia because of poor liver reserves of glycogen.
- Children have a large-surface area and lose heat quickly.
- Children may be insecure or embarrassed if they feel they are not dressed adequately.

### Care during transportation
- Care must be taken to maintain the body temperature especially if the child will be exposed to cold environments. It may be possible to transfer a small baby in a transport incubator, usually used for neonatal transfers, which will provide a heat source.

- Hypoglycaemia should be actively sought. A maintenance source of sugar (IV if necessary) should be available during the journey, as part of the fluid regime. Particular care should be taken with babies who are disconnected from any long-standing sugar source for the journey as they may have relative hyperinsulinism. This includes peritoneal dialysis fluid (especially high-dextrose concentrations) which is often discontinued for convenience during transfer.

## PARENTS

Parents should be regarded as an integral part of the child/doctor relationship and must be kept informed of all developments at all times. A frequent question is whether to allow a parent to travel with the child. This is of great emotional benefit to the conscious child and, in an ideal world, the answer is undeniably 'yes'. Nevertheless, space constraints may make this impractical, particularly if an emergency occurs en route. If parents do not accompany the child, ensure that

- they have a means of travelling to the receiving unit,
- they have clear directions to the receiving unit and the ward,
- they are instructed that, under no circumstances, should they attempt to follow an ambulance that is using blue lights and sirens,
- if they cannot go to the receiving unit themselves, they understand clearly to what ward the child will be admitted and they have the telephone number of the ward.

## NEONATAL TRANSFERS

Many of the principles of paediatric transfer are applicable to this age group but there are some additional differences (Table 8.3).

**Table 8.3    Useful paediatric data**

| To estimate weight (in kg) | 5 months | Double birthweight |
|---|---|---|
| | 12 months | Treble birthweight |
| | 1–9 years | (Age + 4) × 2 |
| | 7–12 years | Age × 3 |
| Endotracheal tube sizes | Premature babies | 2.5 mm |
| | Normal neonates | 3.0 mm |
| | Otherwise | (Age/4) + 4 mm internal diameter |
| | Approximate size | Diameter of nostril |
| Drugs | Epinephrine | 10 μg/kg (0.1 mL 1 in 10,000) |
| | Atropine | 20 μg/kg (maximum 0.5 mg) |
| | Lidocaine | 1 mg/kg (0.1 mL of 1%) |
| Defibrillation | 2 → 4 J/kg | |

It is usual for a paediatrician or neonatologist trained in neonatal transportation to transfer the baby along with a neonatal intensive care nurse.

## Pathology

These babies most commonly require transfer to a specialist unit for the following reasons:

- Complications associated with prematurity.
- Complications associated with delivery such as birth asphyxia or meconium aspiration.
- Surgery – This includes problems such as diaphragmatic hernias, tracheo-oesophageal fistulae, gastroschisis and necrotizing enterocolitis. Many babies are now transferred in utero following antenatal diagnosis.
- Congenital heart disease – the management of complex severe congenital heart disease is very specialized and may involve the use of alprostadil to keep the ductus arteriosus open. Alprostadil can cause apnoea and these babies must be sedated, intubated and ventilated prior to transfer.

Oxygen concentrations should be tailored to the individual needs of the patient because of the effect oxygen has on the adult/foetal circulation balance.

- Other medical congenital or acquired problems, such as hydrops foetalis and renal failure.

In all cases, the management of the baby before and during transfer must be discussed in detail with the receiving unit (preferably consultant to consultant). Treatment which needs to be initiated prior to and during transport may be complex and specific to the disorder.

### Oxygen carriage – a special problem of air transport

HbF has a greater affinity for oxygen than its adult counterpart, hence, a lower $PO_2$ is required to bind a given amount of oxygen. In other words, oxygen is bound more avidly, but results in less liberation in the tissues. The lower $PO_2$ in an aircraft cabin therefore facilitates oxygen delivery to the baby, but hinders its release into the baby's tissues (i.e. HbF and altitude both shift the oxygen dissociation curve to the left). See Figure 7.6.

### Equipment

*The transport incubator*
The transport incubator is the minimum essential piece of equipment for carrying a small sick baby (Figure 8.1). It may be a simple enclosure with battery supply to provide heating and lighting when disconnected from a mains source, whilst more complex versions have a small integral oxygen-powered ventilator and monitoring.

*Neonatal intensive care unit (NICU) equipment*
Sophisticated neonatal retrieval services generally have something much more akin to an 'ICU on a trolley' providing some or

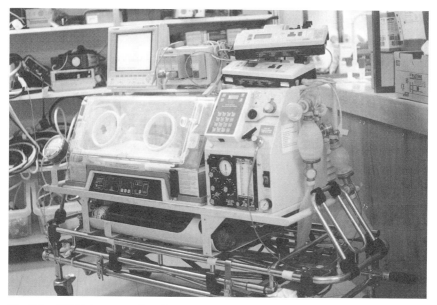

Fig 8.1    NICU transport incubator.

all of the following:

- Incubator with thermostatically controlled heat source.
- Ventilator (of a quality which may be found in a NICU) with humidifier.
- Oxygen and air compressor with oxygen blender.
- Suction aspirator.
- Syringe pumps as required.
- Comprehensive battery system, although most should be capable of using the ambulance battery in transit (and may be compatible with some aircraft electrical systems).
- Monitoring equipment:
    - ECG,
    - inspired oxygen monitor,
    - pulse oximeter,
    - transcutaneous oxygen and $CO_2$,
    - non-invasive /invasive BP monitoring,
    - peripheral/core temperature.

- Drawers containing all necessary equipment for emergencies including chest drains, umbilical venous catheters, endotracheal tubes and resuscitation drugs.
- Occasional equipment such as extra-corporeal membrane oxygenation may be available as part of an extremely specialized retrieval service. Nitric oxide therapy during transport has also been described.

In some countries, dedicated ambulances are equipped specifically for carrying these systems and the retrieval staff. These vehicles may have additional features such as a resuscitaire for emergency procedures that may occur en route.

Neonatal intensive care trolleys are extremely heavy to lift and thought must be given to loading before the ambulance arrives. In an emergency two planks of wood acting as a slope up to the back of the vehicle may suffice if a hydraulic system is not available, but only if used with great care. A final word of warning – some aircraft doors are too narrow, or the angles inside too tight to accommodate these cumbersome incubators. It is important to ensure that any aircraft to be used to transport an incubator is suitable for the purpose.

## FURTHER READING

Advanced Life Support Group (1999) Prehospital Paediatric Life Support. BMJ Publishing Group: London.

Atkins DL, Kerber RE (1994) Paediatric defibrillation: current flow is improved by using 'adult' electrode paddles. Pediatrics 94(1); 90–93.

Barry IW, Ralston C (1994) Adverse events occurring during interhospital transfer of the critically ill. Arch Dis Child 71: 8–11.

Cunningham MD, Smith FR (1973) Stabilization and transport of severely ill infants. Pediatr Clin North Am 20: 359–366.

Dobrin RS, Block S, Gilman JI, Massaro TA (1980) The development of a paediatric emergency transport system. Pediatr Clin North Am 27: 633–646.

Doyle E et al. (1992) Transport of the critically ill child. Br J Hosp Med 48: 314.

Macnab AJ (1991) Optimal escort for interhospital transport of paediatric
emergencies. J Trauma 31: 205–209.

Martin TE, Rodenberg HD (1996) Aeromedical Transportation: A Clinical Guide.
Avebury: Aldershot.

Morse TS (1969) Transportation of critically ill or injured children. Pediatr Clin
North Am 16: 565–571.

Office of National Statistics (1997).

Paediatric Intensive Care Society (1996) Standards for Paediatric Intensive Care.
Saldatore: Bishops Stortford.

Robb HM, Hallworth D, Skeoch CH, Levy C (1992) An audit of a paediatric
intensive care transfer unit. Br J Intens Care 2: 37–39.

Smith DF, Hackel A (1983) Selection criteria for paediatric critical care transport
teams. Crit Care Med 11: 10–12.

# 9

# International repatriation

International travel is well within the pocket of most people and a certain amount of illness and trauma among travellers is only to be expected. Despite the travelling public's fears, very few fall ill as a result of exotic or tropical diseases.

- There is a normal incidence of illness in any population:
  - those with known chronic illness,
  - those with unexpected acute illness.
- Trauma is common in holidaymakers:
  - driving on unfamiliar, badly repaired roads without seat belts;
  - motorcyclists declining to wear crash helmets;
  - over-exuberance with alcohol (a major cause of swimming, diving, and other accidents);
  - specific holiday activities such as skiing, scuba diving, and parasailing.

Repatriation is expensive and beyond the means of most travellers. It is usually a matter for travel insurers but insurance companies rarely have the expertise in medical matters. The actual work of repatriation is contracted to a medical assistance organization in which doctors and nurses form part of a team which decides on

- the urgency of repatriation,
- the mode of transport (dedicated air ambulance, air taxi, charter, or scheduled airliner),
- the type of medical escort (nurse, doctor, specialist) or team,
- any special equipment or procedures required,
- the destination hospital (or home).

The medical assistance doctor has a number of responsibilities, some of which he shares with his nursing and operations colleagues to

- obtain regular medical reports on patients who require assistance,
- complete repatriation and airline medical information forms (MEDIFs) and to liaise with accepting medical team and family practitioner,
- assign and brief the inflight medical escort or team,
- arrange hospital admission or GP referral near the patient's home.

## MEDICAL ASSISTANCE

The medical team, headed by a senior doctor, must have certain skills and knowledge which are unique to the aeromedical arena:

- collate and co-ordinate medical information
    - the medical reports from overseas hospital,
    - medical regulations of the major airlines,

- – guidelines and procedures established by national regulatory bodies,
- – guidelines and procedures of the medical assistance company;
- liaison with hospital specialists, GPs and other agencies;
- possess a good working knowledge of the physical, physiological, and psychological stresses of flight;
- be able to assess and decide upon each patient's fitness to fly;
- co-ordinate arrangements for a safe, acceptable, and comfortable repatriation.

## Medical reports

Good, clear clinical information about the patient is essential. Some overseas referring doctors give excellent reports, but it is occasionally necessary to question medical decisions. In some countries, the treatment of tourists is a lucrative trade, and unnecessary treatments or admissions and delayed discharges are unfortunately common. However, it is best to avoid antagonizing the overseas doctors, since they supply the 'fitness to fly' certificates demanded by the airlines. If they refuse, the patient is grounded. These certificates are essential bureaucracy for many airlines but usually have no real clinical value.

## Urgent repatriation

Urgent repatriation or relocation may be necessary if a case is deemed 'serious' for medical, logistical, or financial reasons (Table 9.1). There are at least four criteria for moving patients urgently (Table 9.2). All assume an immediate requirement for a treatment or procedure that is not available locally and which cannot be brought quickly to the patient. Actual travel details will depend on

- patient's suitability (fitness) for transport,
- medical clearance from the airline,

**Table 9.1    Patients considered to be 'serious'**

| | |
|---|---|
| Medical | Any patient who<br>• is intubated and/or ventilated<br>• would be admitted to an ICU, CCU, or SCBU, with the exception of those with uncomplicated myocardial infarct<br>Patients with<br>• spinal cord injury<br>• subarachnoid haemorrhage<br>Moribund patients |
| Logistic | When the medical facilities are sub-standard and the patient needs transportation to another country for adequate treatment |
| Financial | Any case where the medical fees are rising excessively |

**Table 9.2    Criteria for urgent repatriation**

The condition must be life- or limb-threatening

The patient must be fit enough to survive the physical, physiological, and psychological stresses of flight

A suitably qualified, equipped, and insured doctor and/or nurse (as appropriate) is available to escort the patient

Arrangements have been made for the patient to be collected by ambulance from the destination airport and transferred immediately to the receiving hospital

- flight availability,
- availability of required aircraft seating,
- availability of medical personnel and appropriate equipment,
- positioning flights for medical escorts.

## Repatriation documentation

Most major airlines list their regulations on medical fitness for flight. These rules are advisory, not absolute, but any deviations must be discussed with the medical personnel of the airline concerned. The MEDIF is the interface between the assistance company and the airline. It is important to give as much clinical

Table 9.3    Accepted indications for upgrading of seats
(More than one indication must apply)

| To business class | Within 3 weeks of<br>• major illness (e.g. myocardial infarct)<br>• major operation (e.g. laparotomy)<br>• multiple trauma<br>Age over 60 years<br><br>Duration of<br>• flight over 5 h<br>• travel over 9 h<br>Space needed for medical or nursing care<br>Urgent need for repatriation and lower-class seating not available |
|---|---|
| To first class | If the patient would otherwise be on a stretcher and needs to lie down for a large proportion of the journey, *but*<br>• patient must be continent and able to walk to the wheelchair<br>• no requirement for screening or special privacy |

information as possible, and accurately describe the patient's current condition. It is pointless to mislead airline medical staff. Inflight problems associated with falsification of the MEDIF will soon evaporate the trust between organizations, and future repatriations will suffer.

Logistic details are equally important, for instance when indicating the need for stretcher, wheelchair or upgraded seating. The decision may be influenced by the age and general condition of the patient, and by the estimated flight duration (Table 9.3). Stretchers take up nine seat positions (plus seats for the aeromedical team and accompanying relative) and availability at short notice can be a problem. Oxygen requests can also cause concern. Some airlines do not permit cylinders onboard their aircraft, others charge for use of their own cylinders (which may not be clinically suitable), and most will not yet accept liquid oxygen (LOX), which is considered 'dangerous air cargo'.

## Deciding on the mode of travel

### Air ambulance flights

Air ambulances may be defined as dedicated aircraft used only for the transport of serious cases. They inevitably involve the transfer of very ill patients between hospitals, usually between ICUs. They are, in effect, flying ICUs, staffed by a mixed nurse/doctor (usually an anaesthetist) team.

### Air taxi flights

An air taxi may be defined as a light aircraft or business jet used for the non-urgent transfer of patients when, for operational or logistic reasons, such means of transport is considered more appropriate than a scheduled flight. The indications for both air taxis and air ambulances are given in Table 9.4.

### Commercial airlines

The standard and quality of airline seats, and seat pitch (leg room), vary between aircraft and between airlines. In some

| Table 9.4 | Indications for air ambulances and air taxis |
|---|---|
| Air ambulance | Patient requires ventilation or invasive monitoring |
| | Patient is refused carriage by an airline because of a condition which may be a danger, disruptive or offensive to other passengers |
| | Any other reason for failure of medical clearance by the airline (e.g. oxygen requirements) |
| | Urgent need for repatriation (e.g. in serious cases when local facilities are poor) |
| Air taxis | If a scheduled or charter flight is not available (e.g. because of infrequent services) |
| | When scheduled aircraft facilities are inadequate (e.g. no stretcher capability) |
| | When there is no major airport in the vicinity. Air taxi aircraft can operate into/out of small airfields |
| | Occasionally it is cheaper and easier to use an air taxi than to organize road transportation and/or a sea crossing |

cases, economy seats may vary little from business-class seats on the same airline, or may actually be better than business-class seats on an alternative carrier. In 'double decker' aircraft (such as the Boeing 747), patients should always be accommodated on the lower deck.

## INFLIGHT AEROMEDICAL ESCORTS

The role of the inflight team is not limited to the medical and nursing care of patients while airborne. There are many stages to a successful international repatriation (Table 9.5).

### Pre-flight

The successful assignment starts with good communication and planning. Pre-flight briefing should include the

- patient's clinical details;
- latest medical report;
- equipment and medications to be carried;
- travel details:
  - airports of departure and arrival (and these may differ for the outbound and inbound sectors of the assignment),
  - check-in and departure times,
  - airline and flight details,
  - type of aircraft,
  - requirements for passports, visas, and other special documents,
  - information on the ground ambulance connections at either end of the transfer;
- details of the destination hospital and receiving team.

When satisfied that logistic arrangements are the best that can be made, the medical escort(s) must ensure that all necessary

**Table 9.5   Logistic stages in repatriation assignments**

| | |
|---|---|
| Pre-flight | Medical briefing |
| | Visas, passports, and medical documentation |
| | Suitable equipment, checked, and prepared |
| | Journey to airport, tickets, check-in formalities |
| | Equipment to be kept as hand baggage |
| Outbound | Telephone base office |
| | Adequate rest |
| Patient collection | Handover, notes, reports, investigations, X-rays/scans, and translations |
| | Patient's baggage and personal documentation |
| | Arrangements for accompanying relatives |
| | Transfer to ambulance and compatibility of equipment |
| Airport | Loading, and lifting |
| | Stretchers, wheelchairs, and seats in aircraft |
| | All equipment in cabin and best use of confined space |
| En route | Airborne sectors and sector times |
| | Time zone changes |
| | Stop-overs and facilities |
| | Potential for diversions |
| | Time and temperature at destination |
| | Emergency funds (suitable currencies) |
| Arrival | Airport arrival formalities |
| | Transfer to ambulance and compatibility of equipment |
| | Length of road journey |
| | Total out-of-hospital time |
| Destination hospital or home | Handover to receiving medical team or family practitioner |

equipment is thoroughly checked and prepared prior to leaving the base office. This includes portable oxygen supplies, medications, fluids, special dietary requirements, and other consumables that will be needed for the entire transfer.

## Outbound

Depending on the length of the outbound leg, and the time of arrival, the inflight team may wish to travel directly to see the patient, even if the return flight is not until the following day. This is the time to resolve any problems, not when the ambulance is waiting to take the patient to the airport.

## Patient collection

### Handover

The quality of the handover from the referring team can be extremely variable. It may be very thorough with medical reports already translated and typed, and copies of the investigations and radiographs included, or only the briefest of verbal handovers, mediated through an interpreter. Often, the referring team will have little knowledge of the limitations and dangers of the flight environment, and it remains the escort's duty to ensure that the patient is fit to travel. Finally, if required by the airline, a certificate of fitness to fly must be completed and included in the medical notes.

### Packaging

Patients must be adequately prepared and 'packaged' for movement between hospital bed and both ground and air vehicles. All lines, tubes, and other medical paraphernalia must be functioning and secure before departure. At this stage, the patient will be transferred to the inflight monitoring devices and equipment, although advantage should be taken of any offer from the referring team or ambulance, to supply oxygen or other consumables for the journey to the airport. Similarly, it is always advantageous when the referring hospital can supply any essential medications, although proper planning should ensure that the inflight team carry all essential items overseas.

### Logistics

If luggage is to be placed in the aircraft hold, documents, medications, and any other items needed in flight must be taken as hand baggage. A small selection of local currency may also be necessary to pay for telephone calls, reading materials, snacks, and so on. Stop-overs in endemic areas may require special immunization or prophylaxis arrangements and, finally, the patient must be dressed or wrapped for the coldest environment, whether it be at the point of origin, destination, or in the aircraft.

## Airport

### Embarkation

Patients are usually boarded before able-bodied passengers and offloaded last. Although most international airports now embark passengers via enclosed walkways or piers, smaller airfields still rely on external stairs. An elevator specially designed for the aircraft is preferable for loading stretchers and wheelchairs and for ambulant patients who cannot climb stairs (Figure 9.1).

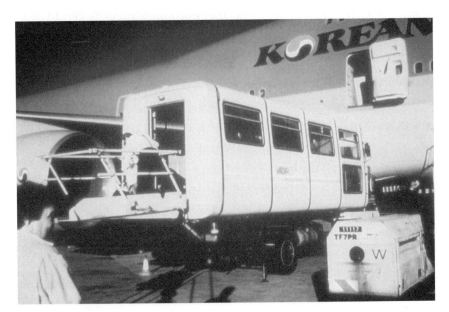

Fig. 9.1   Embarkation is best achieved by means of an elevator.

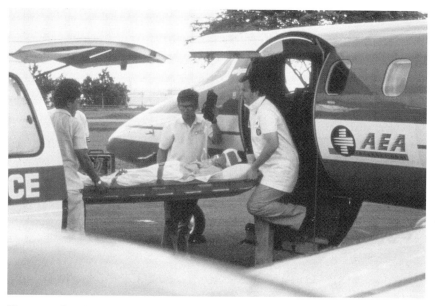

Fig. 9.2   Loading a stretcher onto an air ambulance. Note the difficulty with access and lifting.

Air ambulances suffer the disadvantage of small doors, and it may be impossible to load a stretcher without some degree of tilt which can be frightening for the patient and difficult for the loaders (Figure 9.2).

*Stretchers*

Most major airlines supply stretchers which are usually sited at the rear of the cabin, but only the most modern have back-rests. Extra pillows may be required for those who need, or wish, to sit up. There is continuing debate about whether the patient should lie with the head or foot towards the front of the aircraft but there is no good evidence for any physiological advantage of one over the other in haemodynamically unstable or head-injured patients. Most stretchers are fixed to existing seats, but some aircraft can be fitted with special frames secured to conventional seat mountings on the cabin floor. These frames can accommodate up to three stretchers stacked from floor to ceiling. Curtains are often provided, but usually allow little privacy and cause difficulty in access to the patient and equipment.

### Prior to take-off

Patients must be securely restrained and equipment which is not in immediate use should be stowed. Stretcher patients will need to be screened from the inquisitive eyes of other passengers, and the aeromedical escort must take note of the aircraft safety briefing and the location of emergency exits.

## En route

Although much of the hard work has been done once the patient is onboard, attention must not waiver from the supervision of the patient. Good nursing and medical care must continue and there remains the ever-present possibility of an inflight incident. Medical emergencies may be caused or exacerbated by the flight environment and their management may include descending the aircraft to a lower altitude or, in an extreme, diverting to a nearby airfield. Clearly, the flight crew will be reluctant to divert unless it is absolutely essential. In coming to the decision, the inflight escort must ask where the patient's needs can best be met. If the aircraft's medical team is more skilled and better equipped than the nearest hospital, then clearly there is no advantage in a diversion. When flying over oceans or vast stretches of wilderness, the luxury of a diversion may not be an option. It may be more appropriate to turn back rather than to fly on. There may be other considerations, such as inhospitable regimes or outright warfare in the nearest country, or there may be legal or political implications if the aircraft is diverted. The aircraft captain must be the best judge on these matters.

## Arrival

When safely arrived at the destination airfield, patients will appreciate being taken smoothly through the arrival formalities and, for the severely ill, disembarkation directly on to an ambulance is the rule. The medical assistance company will notify the receiving hospital of the patient's impending arrival, and a bed will have been booked. This speeds the admission procedure and allows a timely handover. As well as the medical notes and investigations collected from the referring hospital, a transfer document should be completed, annotating the travel details and information on any treatments or untoward incidents that occurred in flight. When the receiving team accepts the patient, the inflight escort may return to the base office, being sure to take all items of equipment and unused consumables. Medical waste and used sharps should be correctly disposed of at the receiving hospital. On return to the base office, a copy of the transfer document should be placed on file and all equipment returned and replenishment arranged, ready for the next assignment.

## FURTHER READING

Fairhurst RJ (1992) Health insurance for international travel. In: Dawood R (ed.) Travellers' Health (3rd edn). Oxford University Press: Oxford.

Martin TE (1993) Transportation of patients by air. In: Harding RM, Mills FJ (eds) Aviation Medicine (3rd edn). BMJ: London.

Martin TE, Rodenberg HD (1996) Aeromedical Transportation: A Clinical Guide. Avebury: Aldershot.

Preston FS (1988) Commercial aviation and health – general aspects. In: Ernsting J, King PF (eds) Aviation Medicine (2nd edn). Butterworth: London.

# 10

# Equipment and monitoring

## GENERAL REQUIREMENTS

There is a wide choice of portable medical equipment available, but not all is compatible with the transport environment. Equipment must be suitable for the role, but also able to withstand the stresses of transport. It must be

- accurate,
- reliable,
- dependable without loss of accuracy in thermal extremes and variations in humidity,
- compact,
- lightweight,
- rugged enough to withstand the stresses of accelerations and vibration,
- resistant to pressure changes, if used in aircraft.

## ELECTRICAL EQUIPMENT

Electrical items must be battery powered to avoid the need for vehicle compatibility, especially in aircraft where there is wide variability in electrical systems but few access points to power. Although most ground ambulances predictably use a 12 V system, large passenger carrying aircraft generally operate a 110 V alternating current system, whereas most helicopters and light aircraft use a 28 V direct current supply. Inverters (which convert the electrical supply to 110–240 V alternating current) are needed for equipment which is not capable of independent battery operation. Whatever the vehicle, it must have the capacity to generate enough electrical power to support the simultaneous operation of all onboard equipment (both medical and operational), but any item which leaves the vehicle with the patient must have an independent power supply. Battery life is influenced by charge state and temperature and it is important that adequate power is available for the duration of the entire mission, with sufficient reserves for unexpected delays. Spare charged batteries must always be readily accessible.

## OXYGEN SUPPLIES AND EQUIPMENT

Spare oxygen cylinders must be available for gas-powered machines so that unexpected delays will not use up oxygen necessary for the patient's respiratory requirements. The usual advice is to carry a sizeable reserve – twice the calculated requirement. LOX is an alternative to bulky and heavy oxygen cylinders:

- LOX converters are lightweight insulated containers which may contain up to 25 L of liquid.
- Flow rates are adequate to power ventilators, suction devices and membrane oxygenators without the need for heavy-reducing valves and regulators.
- One litre of LOX stored at $-180°C$ will yield over 800 L of gaseous oxygen.
- The expansion rate is almost seven times greater than pressurized gas in conventional cylinders (at 1800 psi).

- Insulation is imperfect and if oxygen is not being used the gradual rise in temperature causes excess gas production, and pressure within the container increases.
- A relief valve eventually vents this excess so, when calculating oxygen requirements, adjustments must be made to compensate for the fall in oxygen content which starts to occur about 10 h after LOX cylinders are filled.

An alternative method of obtaining high concentrations of oxygen is to generate oxygen by the use of molecular sieves to adsorb nitrogen in compressed air:

- The oxygen generator enriches the oxygen content of air as nitrogen is removed.
- Almost 100% FIO$_2$ is possible, but flow rates are insufficient for gas-driven devices.
- Supplemental cylinders or LOX stores should be carried to cope with faster flow rates and the danger of compressor failure.

Compressed air may be used when high-oxygen concentrations are not required, e.g. to supply incubators during neonatal transfers. Venturi devices can be employed to entrain air for adults requiring intermittent positive pressure ventilation at low or moderate oxygen concentrations, but care must be made to ensure that the patient's oxygen requirements are being satisfied.

## PREHOSPITAL TRANSPORT

In addition to obvious diagnostic and therapeutic medical machinery, items needed by EMS operators include:

- personal safety and rescue items (such as helmets, protective clothing, and metal cutters),

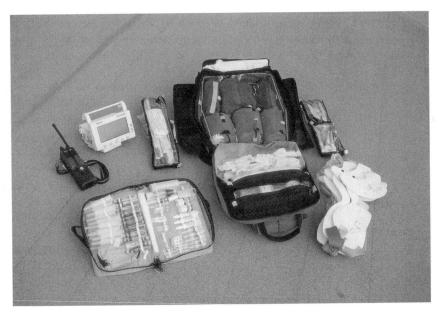

Fig. 10.1   Typical EMS 'snatchbag' equipment.

- ambulance equipment (such as immobilization and extrication devices, stretchers, splints, and blankets),
- communication devices (radio transceivers and mobile telephones).

The minimum amount of diagnostic and therapeutic equipment (Figure 10.1) should include:

- defibrillator with ECG monitor (or a separate monitor),
- pulse oximeter,
- non-invasive BP monitor,
- suction aspirator,
- mechanical ventilator,
- all equipment necessary to safely perform any procedure recommended in the advanced cardiac life-support (ACLS) and prehospital trauma life-support (PHTLS) protocols (Figure 10.2).

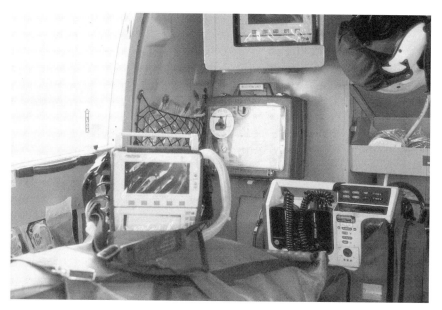

Fig. 10.2    Typical EMS monitoring and therapeutic devices.

Equipment used in out-of-hospital environments must be:

- high visibility,
- water resistant,
- able to withstand the ingress of dust, sand, and salt spray,
- rugged enough to survive a drop from at least 1 m on to any face, side, or corner, without affecting function, accuracy, or reliability.

## INTERFACILITY TRANSPORT AND REPATRIATIONS

Equipment for secondary and tertiary transfers may range from a minimal resuscitation kit for an uncomplicated postoperative or post-infarct repatriation, to a full intensive care capability for critical care patients (Figure 10.3). It is important that all items provide maximum function at minimum cost, size, and weight. Ambulance Trusts, air ambulance organizations, and medical

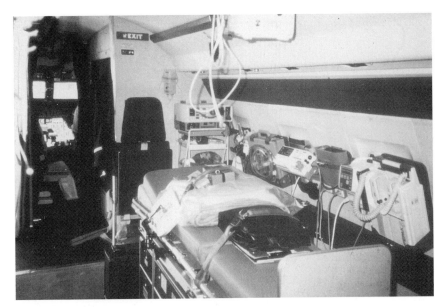

Fig. 10.3    Intensive care kit for a critical care transfer.

assistance companies should keep lists of recommended minimum equipment for the different categories of patients within
their sphere of operations. Further items may be needed depending on information received prior to setting off on the mission.
Good planning may prevent a catastrophe during the transfer.

## CARE OF EQUIPMENT

All electrical, electronic, pneumatic, and mechanical items must
be properly maintained under a servicing schedule in accordance
with the manufacturer's recommendations and must be thoroughly checked before and after any mission. Used consumables
must be replaced, and items fouled or infected must be washed
and disinfected or sterilized before being returned to the medical
store room. Items may be needed urgently for the following mission, and the next team must be spared the task of replenishing
and cleaning equipment before departure.

Equipment for use in aircraft must be checked, tested, and cleared for used by the relevant national aviation authority. Items may prove hazardous in terms of

- spurious electromagnetic fields which interfere with radio and navigation avionics,
- loose object risk during turbulence or emergency landings.

In the UK, all fixed equipment onboard civilian aircraft must be approved by the Civil Aviation Authority (CAA). In principle, portable equipment must also be approved before use, although it is understood that some items may be required at short notice and a common-sense attitude must prevail. Helicopters used in the primary transfer role are a typical example, and Table 10.1 lists the recommendations of the Royal Society of Medicine working party on minimum standards of equipment in medical helicopter systems.

Table 10.1 Recommendations of the Royal Society of Medicine working party on minimum standards of equipment in medical helicopter systems

| Adult | Neonatal |
|---|---|
| Positive pressure ventilation | Transport incubator |
| Pulse oximeter | Temperature monitor |
| BP measurement | Neonatal ventilator |
| ECG | Pulse oximeter or Umbilical |
| Defibrillator | artery oxygen monitor |
| Suction device | BP measurement |
| Oxygen supply | ECG |
| Intubation equipment | Suction device |
| IV fluid equipment | Oxygen supply |
| Drugs for resuscitation | Air supply |
| | Intubation equipment |
| | Drugs for resuscitation and |
| | continuing management |

## SPECIFIC REQUIREMENTS

### Auscultation

Stethoscopes are virtually useless in and around vehicles, especially aircraft and helicopters. Auscultation of the heart and Korotkoff sounds become impossible. Breath sounds are also obscured, making assessment of respiratory status and endotracheal tube placement difficult. Doppler devices can assess blood flow and detect the presence of foetal heart sounds, but little can be done to improve chest auscultation. Good clinical acumen and monitored variables such as oxygen saturation and end-tidal $CO_2$ are essential. Impedance methods of detecting changes in thoracic volume are useful for assessing ventilation.

Be familiar with the alarm systems on the equipment. Audible attention-getters are usually better than visual alarms but vehicle noise limits their reliability. Visual systems are probably safer although suspending them can lead to disaster and visual scanning techniques must be perfected. Unfortunately, long-term scanning and concentration on multiple monitoring devices is fatiguing, and alertness (the time to respond to an alarm) may be impaired.

### Monitoring

Electronic monitoring devices need to be easily accessible, readable in both dim lighting and bright sunlight, accurate, and reliable. With few exceptions, the monitoring of physiological trends is usually of more value than point measurements. As a general rule, it is better to base assessments on the information combined from monitored variables and clinical acumen, rather than rely on monitor measurements in isolation.

#### ECG
Cardiac rhythm is usually monitored by an oscilloscope built into a defibrillator, but small stand-alone battery-powered monitors

are also available, as are multi-function devices, such as the Propaq series. Some machines have the capability of running a rhythm strip, or even a full 12-lead ECG, and some patients may require 24 h ambulatory tape monitoring en route.

### BP

BP can also be monitored on the Propaq, or by stand-alone devices, such as the Dynamap (limb cuff) or Finapres (finger cuff). Invasive arterial and pulmonary BP can also be monitored.

### Temperature

Body temperature may be measured using cutaneous sensors (especially useful for neonatal and burn patients), or body core probes (oesophageal and rectal) and displayed on the Propaq or similar devices. Alternatively, infrared tympanic membrane thermometers are small and reliable.

### Oxygen saturation

Pulse oximetry provides an estimate of oxyhaemoglobin saturation, but it is important to be aware of its limitations. The technique works poorly in the underperfused, gives no information about pulmonary ventilation, can be fooled by carboxyhaemoglobin and methaemoglobin, and makes no adjustment for patients with anaemia. Pulse oximetry will work in neonates, but many paediatricians prefer transcutaneous oxygen saturation monitoring in transit.

### Capnography

End-tidal capnography can provide a continuous $CO_2$ waveform which reassuringly indicates correct endotracheal tube placement. In addition, capnography provides a valuable visual disconnect alarm and important information on the effectiveness of circulation or CPR ($CO_2$ will only be detected if cells are metabolizing oxygen and glucose and circulating blood delivers it to the lungs).

*Cardiotocography*
Portable cardiotocography has recently become available and is now routinely used to assess foetal well-being during the transfer of women in late pregnancy and those at risk of premature delivery.

*Arterial blood gases*
Portable blood gas analysers are now available, although there is sparse literature on their use in the transport environment.

### Therapeutic devices

*Cardioverters*
Defibrillators have been used for many years in ground ambulances, although, for safety, usually when the vehicle is stationary. Studies have shown that they may be operated safely inside aircraft and helicopters during flight. Electricity seeks the path of least resistance and, unless the patient and his surroundings are wet, this path will be through the chest. Very small curent leakage and stray electric fields cause no permanent dysfunction of electronic equipment in the vehicle or aircraft.

*Ventilators*
The ideal portable ventilator is a gas-driven device which provides continuous positive airway pressure (CPAP) and a variable inspiration : expiration ratio. An airway pressure gauge acts as a visible alarm to safeguard against disconnection and barotrauma.

*Infusion devices*
IV syringe drivers are smaller, cheaper, and use less power than infusion pumps, and are routinely used in transport.

*Intra-aortic balloon pumps*
These tend to be operated by only a few selected transportation services with experience of critically ill cardiac patients, mostly in USA.

## Incubators

Portable neonatal incubators are commonly used by transport teams (Figure 10.4). They maintain and control a thermally comfortable environment and may include peripheral equipments such as a cardiac monitor, invasive pressure monitors, a ventilator, portable oxygen supply, and suction aspirator. Oxygen saturation, and transcutaneous oxygen and $CO_2$ is usually also available. Capnography is useful in babies weighing over 2 kg. All portable incubators must have independent internal illumination.

## Implanted therapeutic equipment

A rate-responsive cardiac pacemaker may increase its firing rate because of oversensing due to motion and vibration, or because of interference by electromagnetic fields. Implantable defibrillators may also operate spuriously in the presence of strong electromagnetic fields and have even been activated by the transmissions of mobile telephones.

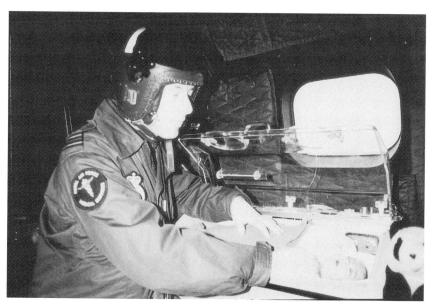

Fig. 10.4   Simple transport incubator used in a military helicopter.

## SPECIFIC AEROMEDICAL PROBLEMS: THE EFFECTS OF GASEOUS EXPANSION

Air or gas trapped within any item of medical equipment or machinery will expand on ascent. This may lead to rupture of part of the equipment, or to damage, failure, or loss of accuracy of measuring or monitoring devices. Table 10.2 lists items of equipment which are susceptible to gas expansion at altitude. Most incidents are predictable, such as follows.

### Air in the cuffs of endotracheal and tracheostomy tubes

Even with a high-volume, low-pressure cuff, air expanding under the influence of lowered ambient pressure is likely to increase transmural pressure across the tracheal wall, and may result in pressure necrosis if it is of sufficient duration and intensity (more than 20 mmHg or 3.0 kPa). Although a pressure limiting pilot balloon will prevent over-inflation at altitude, it cannot prevent a subsequent air leak on descent. The solution is to fill the inflatable cuff with sterile water which, being non-compressible, does not change volume with altitude.

Table 10.2   Equipment susceptible to gaseous expansion

Glass IV fluid bottles
IV administration sets
Pressure bags
Chest drainage bags
NG tubes and other closed drains
Endotracheal tube cuffs
Tracheostomy tube cuffs
Catheter balloons
Sphygmomanometer cuffs
PASG
Air splints

## Splints

Air splints may also expand and contract with altitude. The danger here is either of producing an artificial compartment syndrome or of providing inadequate support and immobilization. The pneumatic antishock garment (PASG), otherwise known as the medical (or military) antishock trousers (MAST) may also cause compartment syndrome at altitude. On descent, relative deflation may cause inadequate pressure support, both to the circulation and to pelvic and lower-extremity fractures. Problems can also occur with loss of solidity of vacuum mattresses at altitude as small volumes of residual air expand.

## IV fluids

Expansion of air in an unvented glass bottle causes a pressure buildup which can lead to shattering. Fluids in plastic bags should be used in preference to those in glass bottles but they still require venting. IV fluids and medications which require exact titration should be regulated by electronic pumps to avoid the artificial increases in flow rate which follows gas expansion and overpressure within the bag.

## Chest drains

Any patient with a pneumothorax should have a functioning tube thoracostomy during flight. If fluid is draining, a valved collection bag should be placed at the outlet of the drain and the bag should be vented when gas expansion occurs. In the absence of fluid, the bag may be safely replaced by a Heimlich valve.

## STANDARDIZATION AND REGULATION OF MEDICAL EQUIPMENT

Table 10.3 illustrates the international standards relevant to medical equipment. New regulations for the approval and monitoring

Table 10.3    International standards for medical equipment

| Description | Standard |
| --- | --- |
| Basic aspects of the safety philosophy of electrical equipment used in medical practice | IEC 513 |
| Medical electrical equipment | IEC 601 |
| Medical suction equipment – electrically powered suction equipment – safety requirements | ISO 10079/1 |
| Environmental conditions and test procedures for airborne equipment (Sections 4–14) | RTCA DO 160C |
| European medical devices directive | 93/42/EEC |

of medical devices were introduced throughout the European Community in 1995. All medical devices must carry a 'CE' mark which signifies that the device has been 'designed and manufactured in such a way that, when used under the conditions, and for the purposes intended, will not compromise the clinical condition or safety of the patient, or compromise the health and safety of the user'.

The Commission Européenne de Normalization has started the task of standardizing land ambulance equipment throughout Europe, but has deferred addressing the complexities of air ambulance equipment because of the difficulty caused by the wide variety of aircraft types and missions.

## INTERNATIONAL DRUG NAMES

The European Union passed legislation that required drug name harmonization by the end of 1999 and some British drug names have changed. In most cases, the difference is only a minor spelling change, such as

- loss of an 'h' (e.g. cholestyramine to colestyramine),
- changing 'i' to 'y' (e.g. amoxycillin to amoxicillin),
- changing 'ph' to 'f' (e.g. clomiphene to clomifene).

| Table 10.4 Changes in British drug names since European harmonization in 1999 | |
|---|---|
| *New Name* | *Old name* |
| Bendroflumethiazide | Bendrofluazide |
| Chlorphenamine | Chlorpheniramine |
| Clomethiazole | Chlormethiazole |
| Dosulepin | Dothiepin |
| Epinephrine | Adrenaline |
| Furosemide | Frusemide |
| Hydroxycarbamide | Hydroxyurea |
| Levomepromazine | Methotrimeprazine |
| Levothyroxine | Thyroxine |
| Lidocaine | Lignocaine |
| Methylthioninium Chloride | Methylene blue |
| Norepinephrine | Noradrenaline |
| Retinol | Vitamin A |
| Tetracosactide | Tetracosactrin |
| Trihexyphenidyl | Benzhexol |

For the foreseeable future, most drugs will be labelled with both the new and the old names. A complete list can be found in the current British National Formulary, but the most commonly affected drugs are listed in Table 10.4.

## FURTHER READING

Anon. (1995) 10th JEMS 1996 Buyers Guide. J Emergency Med Serv Sep: 91–155.

Bristow A et al. (1991) Medical helicopter systems – recommended minimum standards for patient management. J Royal Soc Med 84: 242–244.

British Association of Immediate Care (1995) Equipment Directory. BASICS: Ipswich.

Dedrick DK et al. (1989) Defibrillation safety in emergency helicopter transport. Ann Emergency Med 18(1): 69–71.

Fromm RE, Campbell E, Schlieter P (1995) Inadequacy of visual alarms in helicopter air medical transport. Aviat Space Environ Med 66: 784–786.

Hylton P (1995) What's in a Mark – CE marking for medical devices. Int J Inten Care 2(3): 98.

Joint Formulary Committee (2000) British National Formulary (BNF 40). British Medical Association and the Royal Pharmaceutical Society of Great Britain: London.

Martin TE, Rodenberg HD (1996) Aeromedical Transportation: A Clinical Guide. Avebury: Aldershot.

Martin TE (2000) Fatal delay. Air Ambul Sep: 4–9.

# 11

# Safety at the incident scene

INTRODUCTION

When attending the scene of an accident, personal safety is paramount. Medical and paramedical personnel must take every measure to avoid becoming casualties themselves. The rescuer's priorities are therefore as follows:

- personal safety,
- the safety of the patient,
- the safety of others in the immediate area.

## PERSONAL PROTECTIVE EQUIPMENT

Any rescuer should be suitably attired for the job that they are required to undertake. Clothing should

- be comfortable,
- carry suitable identification ('doctor'/'paramedic', etc.),
- be of high visibility,
- be appropriate for the environment,
- where possible, be fire retardant.

The following areas of the body require special protection:

- Head – protective hard hat or helmet (preferably Kevlar composite) with chin strap.
- Eyes – protective goggles (a visor alone is insufficient when near to operational cutting equipment).
- Ears – ear defenders (where indicated).
- Body – fire retardant overalls; high-visibility waterproof jacket (and trousers if necessary).
- Hands – latex gloves for protection against body fluids and extra gloves for protection against sharp metal, glass etc.
- Feet – strong oil- and acid-resistant boots which protect the feet from crushing.

## DRIVING TO THE SCENE

There are a number of considerations to bear in mind when driving to the scene of an accident, particularly if operating with a blue flashing beacon, where exemption from certain driving regulations may be waived. It is important to remember that a blue light and sirens will not protect the driver either physically or in the eyes of the law, if there is an accident.

### Speed

It is tempting to reach the scene as rapidly as possible, but personal safety and that of other road users must not be jeopardized. A trade-off of safety versus a reasonable response time is necessary. A suitable distance must be kept from the vehicle in front at all times and the driver should always be able to stop within the distance he can see.

### Red mist

Originating on the battlefield, 'red mist' describes a phenomenon where the affected person concentrates on one goal to the exclusion of all else. *This phenomenon is well described in the* drivers of emergency vehicles attempting to reach the scene as rapidly as possible and leads to poor perception of dangers such as adverse driving conditions and lack of awareness of other road users.

## Other road users

When they see an emergency vehicle, members of the public often panic and perform sudden, bizarre, unexpected manoeuvres often in the path of the ambulance or response car. Emergency drivers must be trained to expect such behaviour, for instance in the 'defensive driving' courses provided by the emergency services.

## Type of warning used

On motorways and fast dual carriageways, sirens are less useful and alternating flashing headlights or alternating dipped then undipped headlights may be more effective.

## Doctors

A green flashing beacon on a car identifies the medical practitioner but does not allow exemption from driving regulations in the way that a blue light does. Increasing numbers of immediate care doctors are now equipped with the latter (which must be with the agreement of the chief of police for the area) and can respond in the same way as any other emergency vehicle. It is important that these doctors are properly trained in defensive driving and undergo regular review. When using a blue light, doctors personal cars are sometimes mistaken for unmarked police cars and other road users sometimes brake suddenly in the mistaken belief that they are at risk of being stopped for speeding.

## PARKING AT THE SCENE

There are a number of guidelines for parking at the scene:

- The vehicle should be parked where directed by the police.
- The first vehicle on scene at a road traffic accident (RTA) should protect the accident scene by parking in the 'fend off' position (Figure 11.1). This position will prevent the vehicle being pushed directly into the accident scene if struck from behind, as would occur if the car were parked in line with the accident. It will not, however, offer total protection from oncoming traffic.
- Where emergency vehicles are parked in a line (e.g. at the roadside), the doctor's car is usually parked near to the ambulance which will, in turn, be parked immediately in front of the accident scene (Figure 11.2).

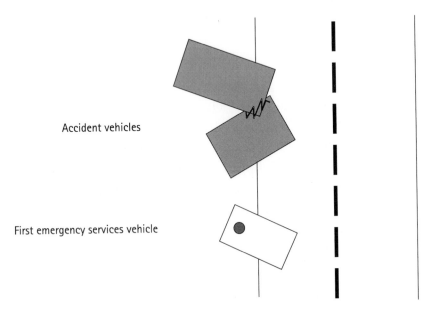

Accident vehicles

First emergency services vehicle

Fig. 11.1   The fend off position.

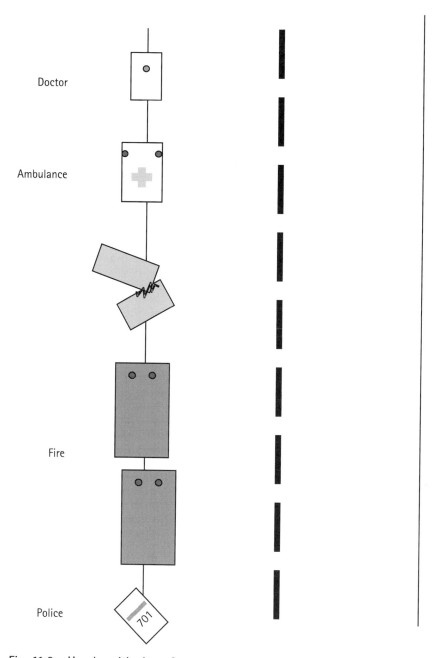

Fig. 11.2   Usual positioning of emergency vehicles at accidents.

## THE ACCIDENT SITE

The police are in overall control at all civilian incidents except where there is unextinguished fire, where the fire service remain in control until the fire is controlled. At any large incident there will be two cordons:

- *The inner cordon*. This is in the immediate vicinity of the incident and the area inside this cordon is known as the bronze area. The area may not be safe and the fire service will control access to this area. In practical terms, the police will hand control of hazards in this area to the fire service. Casualties will generally be removed from the bronze area as soon as possible for treatment, although triage and lifesaving resuscitation may be required at the scene.
- *The outer cordon*. This cordon is controlled by the police and separates the incident scene from the public domain. The area between the inner and outer cordon is known as the silver area and will contain many emergency facilities such as the casualty clearing station and the emergency control vehicles.

Medical personnel should seek the advice of the fire service and the ambulance safety officer (who is responsible for the safety of all medical personnel) regarding entry to and safety within the inner cordon. It is likely that access to this area will be restricted.

## SPECIFIC SAFETY ISSUES

Every type of incident has its own specific safety issues. Some of the more common dangers and situations are outlined below. It must be borne in mind that more that one type of incident may occur at any one event.

## Road traffic accidents

- Beware of other traffic.
- There is a legal requirement regarding the type and quantity of high-visibility clothing to be worn on motorways. It is, however, advisable to wear clothing of a similar high standard of visibility at all RTAs.
- Damaged cars may be physically unstable and occasionally at risk of fire, though this is rare once the engine is switched off.
- Sharp metal and glass fragments are a universal danger.
- There may be a risk of sudden deployment of unexploded air bags.

## Chemical incidents

- GET OUT of the area (go upwind), CALL OUT the fire service and STAY OUT of the area until it is deemed safe by the fire service.
- Be careful of your approach to a known hazardous scene – ensure the access is away from gas clouds, i.e from upwind.
- Be aware of the different chemical identity cards (Kemmler, Hazchem) and methods of gaining first aid advice (Transport Emergency (TREM) Card and CHEMDATA, accessible via the fire service).
- Decontamination of affected individuals is essential and may take priority over the medical needs of the patient. Do not become another victim or allow other rescuers (including the hospital) to endanger themselves by becoming contaminated.

## Railway incidents

- Approved high-visibility clothing is essential, with reflective markings if working in a tunnel.

- Be alert for approaching trains at all times and observe the minimum required distance to maintain the position of safety (varies from 2.75 to 1.25 m depending on the maximum permitted speed of the train).
- Do not cross or walk on any line except at a level crossing unless it is absolutely necessary.
- Overhead electric lines carry a potential of up to 25 kV. Keep well away (at least 2.75 m) from them or anything dangling from them.
- The conductor rail (third rail) carries voltages up to 750 V. Do not cross it unless absolutely essential and then only at protected points. Even when the electricity has been switched of it may take considerable time for the charge to dissipate. 'Fourth' rails, if present should be treated in the same way as 'third' rails.

### Aircraft crashes

- Never enter a live runway or taxiway without permission. Do not proceed directly to an aircraft accident without contacting the airport air traffic control or being escorted by the police or airport authorities.
- Helicopters should not fly directly over the area. They will disturb any foam blanket laid by the fire service and 'stir up' and spread potentially dangerous carbon fibres.
- The inner cordon is tightly controlled by the fire service who are responsible for activities within. Access is strictly limited and safety precautions strictly enforced.
- Certain composite materials used in aircraft construction may produce dust and fibres that may cause both acute and long-term damage to health. If these are present in significant quantity, chemical protection suits will be worn (by the fire service) and chemical incident rules for contamination should be observed.

- Military aircraft have additional hazards such as laser sights and explosives in missiles and in unused ejector seats. Seek advice.
- Stay well clear of working jet engines (at least 8 m).

### Radiation incidents

- Position the vehicle upwind from the incident.
- Contamination depends on the mechanism of exposure – if the exposure is to penetrating radiation there is no risk to the rescuer from the patient, but if there has been external contamination the risk will vary, depending on whether there is ongoing exposure at the scene or simply residual contamination from the patient.
- Before eating, drinking or smoking, the rescuer should be checked by the medical physics department of the hospital to check they have not been contaminated.

### Confined spaces/unstable structures

- If asked to enter such areas (such as underground disasters, house explosions or bomb incidents), check your personal limitations before going in. Panic from claustrophobia in such a scenario will endanger not only your own, but other people's lives. If in doubt, do not go in.
- If you enter such areas be certain you are adequately protected – if the fire service are using breathing apparatus and you are not, you should not be there.
- Be sure you are adequately trained in the potential dangers of the scene and be aware of any emergency procedures.

### Shootings/bombs

- Confirm that the area is safe from further bullets or explosions before entering.
- Obtain police protection if necessary.

- Some detonators are radio controlled and therefore susceptible to radio frequency interference. Do not use a radio, as it may set off an explosion.

## Electrocutions

- Ensure that the electrical source has been switched off before touching the patient.
- It may be necessary to call emergency electrical engineers to cut off a power supply.

Finally, at all incidents, remember that whistle blasts are used by the fire service to indicate that immediate evacuation from the scene is required.

## SAFETY AROUND HELICOPTERS

Doctors, paramedics, and flight nurses working for helicopter emergency medical services (HEMS) may be exposed to a variety of environments and extremes of climate as a part of their daily operations. Flight uniforms and equipment must be

- protective for the accident scene:
  - warm and adaptable enough for extreme temperatures,
  - tough and resistant to 'wear and tear',
  - helmet suitable for use in dangerous scenarios;
- protective for the aviation environment:
  - fire retardant,
  - oil and fuel resistance,
  - helmet suitable for use in helicopters,
  - hearing protection and good communications;
- protective against biological waste
  - gloves,
  - eye protection.

Although helicopter crews work in a hazardous environment, they also bring a hazard (the helicopter) to the scene when they respond. The pilot is often unfamiliar with the landing site and may be distracted by the scene, other emergency service vehicles and by people on the ground. When approaching a difficult confined area, the danger of rotors striking trees, buildings or roadside 'furniture' is a constant threat.

These dangers emphasize that aeromedical personnel must be familiar with specific emergency procedures and safety issues of each aircraft type in use. Once on the ground, however, helicopter landing zones are still inherently dangerous places:

- The most obvious risk is of injury from rotor blades and tail rotors. This danger is heightened during start-up and shut-down of the engines (especially when the wind speed is high), as blades dip lowest to the ground when rotors are slow. Like all passengers and ground staff, medical personnel should approach the aircraft only at the discretion and direction of the captain (or other nominated flight crew), and never from the rear, where there is a danger of tail rotor strikes in most helicopter types.
- Injuries may also occur as debris, dust, sand, snow or spray are propelled through the air by rotor wash.
- These dangers are intensified by increased noise levels (difficulty in hearing warnings), and slippery surfaces found on exposed landing pads.
- All personnel who may interact with HEMS helicopters must be properly educated in patient transfer techniques and landing zone safety, or should keep well clear.

Inappropriate contact with the helicopter also presents a problem. Heated pitot tubes may cause burns if touched immediately after flight, and radio antennas which are capable of high energy dissipation often look like handles and can cause shocks if touched during radio transmission. Finally, aircraft may be damaged by careless behaviour at a landing zone. Ambulances and other vehicles have been known to impact helicopters, usually in the enthusiastic desire to assist with expeditious patient loading.

## FURTHER READING

Advanced Life Support Group (1995) Major Incident Medical Management and Support – The Practical Approach. BMJ: London.

Greaves I, Hodgetts T, Porter K (1997) Emergency Care – A Textbook for Paramedics. Saunders: London.

Hodgetts T, McNeil I, Cooke M (1995) The Prehospital Emergency Management Master. BMJ: London.

Lancashire Fire and Rescue Service and All Lancashire Emergency Response Team (1997) Safety at Scene Course Manual, Lancashire Fire and Rescue Service and All Lancashire Emergency Response Team, International Training Centre, Washington Hall.

Martin TE (1994) Planning medical services for air disasters. In: The Management of Disasters and Their Aftermath. BMJ: London.

# 12

# Medicolegal aspects of patient transport

## INTRODUCTION

The issues of standards of care, consent, liability, documentation, confidentiality, and clinical management guidelines are as important in patient transport as in normal clinical practice. International air ambulance operations are potentially far more complex – the problems of jurisdiction, importation and exportation of drugs, international health regulations, and birth and death in flight, are of additional significance. The operation, and hence the liabilities, of a helicopter emergency medical service in the prehospital environment is similar to that of a ground ambulance.

## STANDARDS OF CARE

The doctor/patient relationship is unique although many of the fundamental obligations and responsibilities of this relationship are shared by nurses and paramedics acting alone during patient transfers. Once a doctor offers advice, he creates a contract, even in the absence of formal mutual consent. After a patient requests diagnostic and therapeutic services, the doctor accepts a duty to provide the appropriate standard of medical care. In the out-of-hospital environment the establishment of a contract is not so obvious. The patient may be unconscious and may not have purposefully and intentionally sought a doctor's advice before the emergency or the transfer actually occurs. However, the duty with respect to standards of care remains the same. It has three components: to exercise a degree of knowledge, skill, and due care, similar to that expected of a reasonably competent practitioner with a comparable background who acts in the same or similar circumstances.

Doctors may have their own self-imposed moral code and are subject to ethical guidelines imposed by professional organizations but, in the UK, there is no legal duty to rescue or resuscitate another person. From the legal standpoint, a doctor who by chance encounters an emergency need not offer his services. However, once treatment is started, a legal duty exists to do all that is reasonable to complete the resuscitation successfully. Some countries have initiated 'Good Samaritan' regulations to encourage potential rescuers to offer aid in emergency situations.

## CONSENT

An assault or battery is committed when there is intentional and unpermitted touching of another person. Medical care in the absence of consent may therefore be considered an assault, but when life is at risk the law presumes that any reasonable person would want to be saved. It infers consent, even when not formally obtained. Adults of sound mind and courts acting on behalf of children and the incapable have the right to refuse treatment, but clearly must be fully aware of the consequences of such refusal. An 'Advance Statement' (Living Will) allows a person, when healthy and of sound mind, to state how he would wish to be treated if unable to express an opinion. Although not legally binding in the UK, these documents are becoming increasingly common among those who wish not to have life prolonged after suffering serious damage with no prospect of normal recovery. Recent human rights legislation is likely to have serious repercussions on how 'informed consent' is achieved, but doctors are advised to inform patients of all significant risks and, preferably, to obtain the patient's verbal and signed consent contemporaneously (although this will not abrogate the patient's right to take future legal action).

## LIABILITY

The responsibilities and obligations of the doctor, nurse, or paramedic are no different than they are in normal everyday practice and no health professional should fear litigation if diligence and due care is exercised during patient management. A successful law suit must prove that the doctor has performed in a grossly negligent manner. Negligence requires the plaintiff to establish four elements:

- the appropriate standard of care, usually by expert medical testimony;
- a breach of that standard;
- a demonstrable injury;
- a causal link between the breach of duty and the claimed injury.

Careless conduct may constitute grounds for legal liability, even though there was no conscious design to do wrong. When negligence is proven, the patient is entitled to invoke the process of law to obtain compensation. However, the UK has not adopted 'No Fault Liability' laws, and injury alone confers no legal rights. The law has no redress without fault attributable to a person.

Any person can be held liable for negligence, but only where there is failure to observe the standard of care which the law requires him to observe in the performance of a duty owed by him to the injured person. Clearly, these standards differ between the professions and, in a team situation, the most senior person may carry responsibility for his juniors. When a doctor is present, final responsibility for the well-being of the patient will be his, although liability may be shared by supervising medical seniors. Relationships between members of the team must be carefully delineated – all are mutually dependent upon each other and good rapport is crucial to minimize potential liabilities.

Medical and paramedical personnel, ambulance operators, and medical directors all face the risk of liability, not only for their own actions, but also for those working under or for them. Normally the employer is vicariously liable for the acts and omissions of an employee but the medical director of an EMS system or ambulance trust may also be deemed responsible for the actions of emergency medical personnel under his supervision. This is the legal concept of respondent superior ('let the master answer', i.e. the 'master' is liable in certain cases for the wrongful acts of his 'servant').

## DOCUMENTATION

A common problem in cases of malpractice liability is the poor standard of documentation. Good notes are essential. They must be

- accurate,
- legible,
- clear,
- concise,
- complete,
- attributable (and signed),
- contemporaneous (timed and dated).

Memory is unreliable and is nothing more than unsubstantiated evidence in court. Alterations to records must be signed and annotated with the date, time, and reason for the correction. Lawyers are understandably suspicious of changes made retrospectively. Dictaphone tapes are not considered legal documents but they can be used for contemporaneous note taking as long as they are transcribed into written form at the earliest opportunity. In the European Community, patients have open access to their written medical documents as well as to computer records. Finally, it is imprudent to write anything which could prove embarrassing if disclosed in court.

*Pre-transfer assessment*   The first entry should identify or exclude problems which may be important to the safe conduct of the transfer. Included at this stage should be the results of any investigations or special examinations necessary before decisions are made on fitness to move, or on the conditions of the transfer.

*Transfer record*   Clear details of the transfer process should be entered, along with a summary at the safe conclusion of the transfer. The following should be annotated:

* mode of transport,
* departure time,
* monitoring and investigations en route,
* treatments and interventions en route,
* incidents and subsequent actions,
* significant interactions with the patient, relatives, or other third parties.

*Handover*   At the destination, in addition to a verbal handover, the medical team should transfer all notes, X-rays, and investigations from the referring hospital, along with the summary which outlines the logistic details of the journey as well as the clinical details described above.

Notes taken during primary missions will inevitably be shorter and specifically relevant to the prehospital emergency situation. Despite the need for brevity, the same considerations must apply, i.e. that they are written in a clear, concise, accurate, and legible manner, appropriately dated and signed, with the timings of the incident, arrival on scene, and arrival at hospital duly noted.

## CONFIDENTIALITY

Patients (or those acting legally on their behalf) must consent to the disclosure of information. However, if disclosure is considered essential and in the best interests of the patient, this must be justifiable later. For instance, the captain of a dedicated air ambulance is usually informed of the general nature of the patient's condition because of any constraints or limitations that it may impose on the operation of the aircraft. Otherwise, patients are entitled to expect that information learned by members of the medical team during the course of the transfer will remain confidential.

## CLINICAL CODES OF PRACTICE

Clinical practice is increasingly being governed by policies, protocols, guidelines, and codes of practice, and there is no doubt that they standardize patient management. Health professionals may be comforted in the belief that adherence to these policies offers some protection against liability but, until the evidential basis for clinical guidelines is confirmed, their legal status remains questionable.

*Clinical guidelines*    Legally validated clinical guidelines are being produced in America to ensure that doctors who comply with them are shielded against liability. Under English law, guidelines and policies are only hearsay evidence because they are written documents and cannot be cross examined. They may be accepted as established standards of care, but are no substitute for expert testimony and an expert witness may be asked whether there is a significant body that rejects them in favour of a different approach.

*'Do Not Resuscitate' (DNR) policies*    There remains a reluctance in the UK and many parts of the world to legislate on DNR issues which are often emotive and carry potential for litigation. Brain death criteria are useful in the ICU scenario but impossible, in the transport environment.

## MEDICOLEGAL ISSUES SPECIFIC TO INTERNATIONAL AEROMEDICAL TRANSFERS

### Jurisdiction

Jurisdiction is defined as the right to administer justice and to apply laws. When an aircraft is in international airspace, the country with jurisdiction may well be disputed, depending on the nature of the incident or situation in question. Jurisdiction may belong to the country

- of manufacture of the aircraft,
- where the airline or carrier is based,
- in which the aircraft is registered (sometimes different from the above),
- where the crew are based,
- most recently overflown,
- most recently departed.

The American population is much more litigious than in other countries and, if an incident occurs on an US registered aircraft, or involves an American patient, an action might be brought in the USA. All medical personnel working in international repatriation would be well advised to be sure of adequate insurance cover for liability in the American courts.

## Licencing to practice

Another unique concern in air ambulance operations is the issue of licencing and professional practice across national borders. There is potential for liability or even criminal action if medical care is given by an aeromedical escort, or under the authority of a medical director, when either is not licenced to practice in the country of patient pickup or delivery. International transfers also raise concerns about visas, border controls, and the carriage of controlled substances.

## Importation and exportation of drugs

Most countries prohibit the importation and exportation of medicines unless they are required for personal treatment or unless import/export authorization has been granted. Annual export licences are available through air ambulance and medical assistance companies so that named individuals can take drugs out of the country and bring them back again if unused. A letter from the medical director (preferably written in the language spoken at the destination or pickup point overseas) explaining the medical nature of the mission may ease problems at immigration and customs. Drugs may appear on controlled lists in some countries but not in others, and it is important to maintain an inventory of all drugs carried and also a record of those actually used during the transfer. The inventory available and the equipment bag should be available for inspection at national borders although problems may still arise. For instance, diamorphine

(*Heroin*), a commonly used drug in the UK, is prohibited in the USA, even for prescribed medical use.

In the UK any registered practitioner can write a prescription for controlled drugs, as long as that prescription is correctly completed with the prescribed dose written in both words and numbers. Controlled drugs in the USA are supplied only if the Drugs Enforcement Agency registration number of the prescribing physician is known. In both countries the doctor is responsible for absolute security of the drugs and an accurate record of their use.

## International Health Regulations

Most countries are signatories to the World Health Organization's International Health Regulations (IHRs), or have adopted their own more stringent regulations. IHRs cover immunization procedures, quarantine methods, and the prevention of transmission of disease and of disease vectors. There are only three diseases which are 'subject to the regulations' and for which special provisions are made:

- cholera,
- yellow fever,
- plague.

A further five diseases are 'under surveillance':

- poliomyelitis,
- influenza,
- malaria,
- louse-borne relapsing fever,
- louse-borne typhus.

Countries are free to add other diseases which may be of local concern. In the UK, the regulations are loose enough to cover 'any other infection or infestation in a person or aircraft arriving or departing' but the list specifically includes:

- lassa fever,
- marburg disease,
- viral haemorrhagic fever,
- rabies.

The transport of patients with active and dangerous contagious diseases should only take place in exceptional circumstances. Consider the risks and benefits very carefully in patients who have an extremely poor prognosis. The difficulties include:

- Airlines will not carry these patients.
- Air ambulance and charter organizations will require daunting and expensive isolation facilities and procedures.
- Safe fumigation and disinfection of aircraft is time consuming, costly and extremely difficult to achieve.
- Innumerable people will be placed at risk.

### Birth and death in flight

Most airlines will refuse to carry terminally ill patients. For those who must travel in their final days, for instance to return home to die, the only solution is usually by private air ambulance. Nevertheless, death may occur unexpectedly during planned aeromedical missions, and may even happen to passengers not being carried as patients (British Airways reported 14 inflight deaths between April 1991 and March 1992; only two of these were patients known to the medical department before departure). When a death occurs in flight, five options present themselves to the aeromedical and flight crews:

- Notify the nearest air traffic control service and land at the designated diversionary airfield.

- Record the exact navigational position at the time of death and return to the point of origin to notify the authorities.
- Record the exact navigational position at the time of death and continue on to the planned destination before notifying the authorities.
- Continue resuscitation attempts until able to divert to a 'friendly' country with the same or similar laws as those which are familiar to the medical and flight crew, and then notify the authorities.
- Continue resuscitation attempts until entering airspace of the planned destination, and then notify the authorities.

The decision is based on local knowledge and which particular jurisdiction has interest in the death. Some countries have laws with regard to the payment of death taxes, or over the distribution of the estate of the deceased. The medical escort must consider the bereaved relatives. Not only will they have the major problem of arranging for the return of the body, but they may also become entangled in complex and expensive legislation. Under such circumstances, there may be a case for continuing resuscitation attempts until the aircraft enters 'friendly airspace', at the planned destination, or at a suitable diversion en route. Decision making is more complicated when the medical escort is not a qualified doctor. In most countries, only medically trained personnel may certify death. In this case the patient cannot be legally dead until certified by a doctor at the next available landing. Whatever decision is taken, the medical escort must keep the captain, his cabin crew and any accompanying relatives fully informed of the actions to be taken, and the justification for these actions.

Births en route are less of a problem. Although most airlines will refuse carriage to any woman over 35 weeks pregnant, labour may be premature and some passengers in the late stages of pregnancy may travel unannounced. Clearly, there are many problems associated with delivery on board an aircraft but, from a legal point of view, the only issue is of nationality and place of registration of birth of the newborn. This, once again, is a problem of jurisdiction.

## PERSONAL ACCIDENT INSURANCE

Under new NHS regulations, additional personal accident insurance to cover incidents occurring outside of hospital cannot be provided by NHS Trusts, and health professionals are strongly advised to acquire appropriate cover. This may be possible through professional organizations.

The Association of Anaesthetists of Great Britain and Ireland and the Intensive Care Society provide insurance for members who escort patients in ambulances, helicopters, aircraft and boats, for both the escorted and staging (or returning) sectors. Accidents while driving personal cars to an emergency are also covered. The key features of the cover are

- up to £1 million per member,
- £5 million limit per vehicle,
- the cover is worldwide,
- protection for usual occupation,
- there is a scale of payouts for injuries that are not fatal,
- private transfers are covered,
- transfers for other organizations, such as HM Coastguard and the RNLI are covered,
- the escort must be a 'passenger' when flying, not a flight crew member,
- the insurance is included as a benefit in the annual subscription at no extra cost.

Insurance cover for injury while on NHS duty is provided from the NHS Injuries and Death Benefit Scheme, but benefits are based on salary and time in post in particular, and are often inadequate, especially for trainees. Health Authorities may have local arrangements but, in general, the inadequacy of cover available from NHS Trusts makes additional personal accident insurance a necessity.

## FURTHER READING

Chapman PJC (1993) Legal aspects of inflight emergencies. In: Harding RM, Mills FJ (eds) Aviation Medicine (3rd edn). BMJ: London.

General Medical Council (1995) The Duties of a Doctor. GMC: London.

General Medical Council (1995) Good Medical Practice. GMC: London.

General Medical Council (1995) Confidentiality. GMC: London.

Hurwitz B (1995) Clinical guidelines and the law. BMJ 311: 1517–1518.

Martin TE, Rodenberg HD (1996) Aeromedical Transportation: A Clinical Guide. Avebury: Aldershot.

Mookini RK (1990) Medical–legal aspects of aeromedical transport of emergency patients. Legal Med pp 1–30.

Mitchell M (1993) Legal ramifications in air medical transport. In: Rodenberg H, Blumen IJ (eds) Air Medical Physician's Handbook AMPA: Salt Lake City.

World Health Organization (1983) International Health Regulations (3rd edn). WHO: Geneva.

# Index